ALZHEIMER'S

We Were There But So Was God!

**Advantage
INSPIRATIONAL**

Gwen Bibber Kimball

ALZHEIMER'S: We Were There – But So Was God! by Gwen B. Kimball

Copyright © 2005 by Gwen B. Kimball
All Right Reserved
ISBN: 1-5975502-9-9
Published by: Advantage Books
                  www.advbooks.com

Library of Congress Control Number: 2005926266

First Printing: May 2005

05 06 07 08 09 10 11   9 8 7 6 5 4 3 2 1
Printed in the United States of America

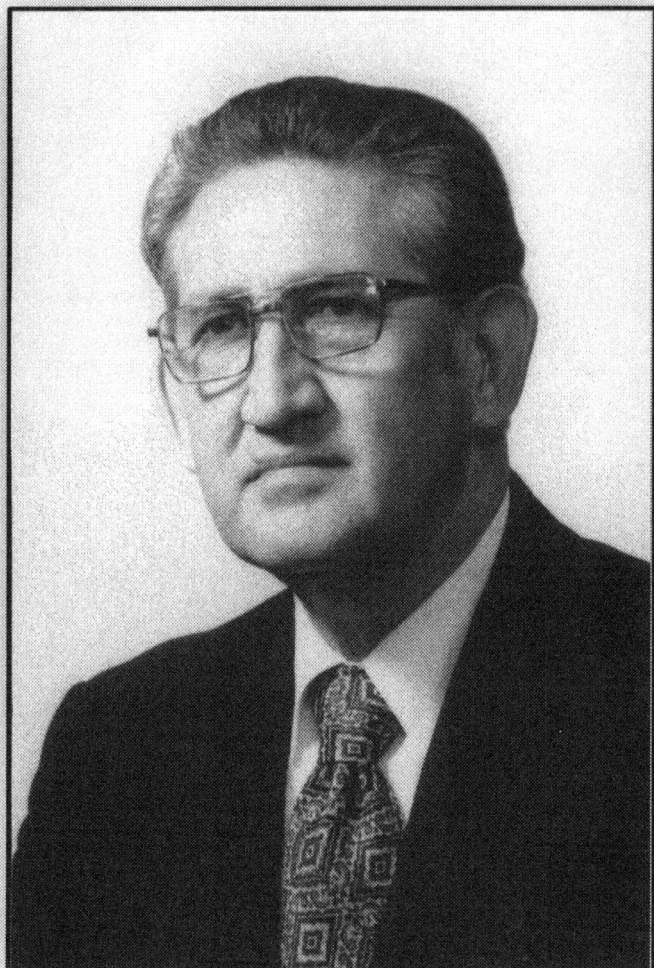

DEDICATION

To my dear husband

Dave Kimball

I dedicate this, our story.

Gwen Bibber Kimball

TABLE OF CONTENTS

FOREWORD

When I was asked to review the manuscript for Gwen Kimball's new book, it was a privilege. When I was subsequently asked to write the foreword for this wonderful volume, it was an unspeakable honor.

I have known Dave and Gwen Kimball all my conscious life. During my childhood "Pastor Kimball" ministered the local church of which we were a part; during my adolescence "Uncle Dave" and "Aunt Gwen" were dear family friends we visited when traveling east; as an adult I was privileged to have Dave perform my wedding ceremony as Alzheimer's Disease, not yet recognized, was insidiously beginning to ravage his mind.

My interest in this book stretches beyond the personal level, however. As a physician, I have cared for countless patients and their families whose world reels from the effects of Alzheimer's Disease.

This affliction is never easy. If it is possible to be more devastating to one person than another, Alzheimer's hits hardest those whose life's accomplishments are mental rather than physical. Of such stock was David Kimball: scholar, teacher, wise counselor. In this book we get a most intimate view of his experiences as he progresses from minor memory problems, to the terrifying realization of what was occurring, to near oblivion.

The condition does not merely affect the individual. The largest burden falls upon the loved ones, the family, the caregiver. Gwen Kimball bares her soul as she recounts the very personal experiences through which she and Dave passed, transporting the reader into their world. The joys, frustrations, and experiences of Divine intervention are felt first-hand while reading their story. Other works I've read focus only on the trials, or only on the victories. Both approaches are equally empty. This account does an outstanding job of presenting an honest, balanced, complete, and personal view of Alzheimer's Disease from the "inside".

For those who are experiencing Alzheimer's Disease with a loved one, this book can be a boon to the spirit. Its reading will undoubtedly draw tears, but its tender tale will be a balm to the soul. I wholeheartedly commend it to your attention.

Mark K. Huntington, MD PhD FAAFP
Ortonville, Minnesota

ACKNOWLEDGMENTS

To our daughters, Midge, Karen and Michelle, who faithfully saw us through this odyssey. Thank you for being there.

Gwen Bibber Kimball

INTRODUCTION

Dave Kimball and I could have chosen to let this Alzheimer's experience be ours alone. Our final seven years together could have been hidden and private, years not shared, not exposed to public view. However, when the number of Senior Citizens is increasing at a rate of three to one over any other age group, and too large a percentage of those either are, or will be, afflicted with Alzheimer's, can the sharing of one couple's struggles be meaningful? We hope so. It is with this hope in mind that we disclose details of our lives that normally would remain entirely personal.

I cry softly as I ask myself questions. When did we last share mutual meaningful love? I can't remember. When did we have our last meaningful discussion? I can't remember. When did we last share a hearty laugh over something that David Kimball recognized as humor? I can't remember that either, along with many other things that faded from our lives long ago.

We came full-circle from whole-hearted love, whole-hearted energy, and whole-hearted purpose, to a firm love-commitment, barely enough energy for each long day, and only one remaining purpose: that of the "one" caring for the "other" until this Alzheimer's thing was over.

It was over on April 27, 2000, when God welcomed Dave to his home in Heaven. No more need for that love-commitment by his caregiver. No more long days and nights of dark despair for the victim. Dave is free.

Chapter 1

TWIGS

The year was somewhere in the early 1990's. Dave wandered across the yard, scanning the ground studiously. In his hand was a collection of twigs — mostly three inches or so long. At first he did this once a day. Then twice. Each day the routine was the same. The number of times increased until finally my mind got the message, and I stood in the window and cried. Here was my college-valedictorian husband, reduced to nothing more mind stimulating than picking up twigs, many of which were so small I would not have even noticed them.

Finally, after several years of wondering, I realized down deep that we had a problem. That realization propelled me into an entirely new phase of my own. I obviously could not stand in the window and cry for the remainder of my life. I must revise my expectations, and I must start adapting to the now, not to what used to be. It all must start with my trying to lay aside his past mental capabilities and accept what were becoming the very simple, routine, almost childlike capabilities of the present.

This was especially hard to do. This man was a retired pastor who had had a keen grasp of Bible Doctrine. He had based his ministry upon teaching. He had made important points of things that escaped my more average mentality and, I suspect, the average mentality of some of his parishoners also. For many years he had taught carefully and well.

When did this condition, which resulted in Dave's being reduced to picking up twigs, actually begin? I have asked myself that question many times. How does one go back and put a finger on the first indications of a personality change, of a lessening of mental acuity, or of memory loss? As one ages, how does one distinguish between normal and abnormal?

As I pondered these questions I recalled incidents as far back as a couple of decades that seemed to indicate that there were problems -- things that pricked my awareness that something was not exactly right. Yet, even that much evidence seemed insufficient to send me on an all-out crusade to determine what in the world was wrong here.

I do remember wondering, vaguely, if there was a test somewhere out there in the medical world that could determine the malfunctioning of a person's mind. But in that day I didn't even know anyone I felt free to ask such a question. The very thought seemed bizarre. I had never yet heard of Alzheimer's.

Furthermore, what of the man? What of David Kimball being subjected to tests to determine his mental competence? For what reason? Perhaps, indeed, just because of some very trivial changes due to the aging process? Better to call it burn-out, stress, anything except there being a problem with someone's brain! I could envision a lowering of Dave's self-esteem and of confidence in his ministry, perhaps for nothing. It all seemed so far-out, preposterous, and even insulting. And besides, he slept well, ate well, dressed impeccably, read a lot. So I tucked the whole subject away, so I thought. But it continued to lurk there in the shadows, and increasingly it reappeared to remind me that all was not right.

Two crises in his life further pointed up the presence of problems. In 1989, open-heart surgery and its recovery period were accompanied by serious mental confusion. In 1991 a single-car automobile accident caused by Dave's deteriorating driving skills resulted in his suffering a neck fracture. Both stays in the hospital required sitters at night to control his anxious and unpredictable behavior which included, after the neck fracture episode, the almost constant removal of his neck brace -- further proof of his inability to reason.

The nursing staff repeatedly reminded him that he must not take his brace off. This was met each time with an apology, an empty smile, and a promise to comply, followed by his predictably trying to remove it again soon after. The style of brace was changed several times in order to find one that he could not remove easily, culminating in one which I called "the contraption." To no avail.

Our Pastor, Ken Nanfelt called me from Dave's bedside one morning to report on how well he was looking. I asked him what he thought of the brace and he replied, "Oh yes, I see it over there on the bedside table." My reply was, "WHAT?!"

I called the nurses' station in a panic and asked them if they were aware that Dave was using his neck brace as a centerpiece for his bedside table. At that point they reinstalled it so securely with tape that I feared we might never get it off, ever again! However, no brace totally prohibited his lifting his chin or turning his head, slightly.

His return home from his hospital stay was not without fear on my part. How could I be sure that his neck brace would be in place every minute, night and day? Damage to the area of this fracture could mean a spinal cord injury with dire results. Butterflies took up almost permanent residence in my stomach.

On several occasions we found him in the garage, chopping wood, brace notwithstanding. My pleading precipitated only anger, which was not characteristic. Our daughter Karen's approach was one of asking him to "indulge her," which he did quite willingly -- until the next time he forgot.

We managed both recovery periods without serious incident, but bouts of depression and decreased memory became the final catalysts in attempting to determine what was happening in the life of Dave Kimball. The suggestion by his doctor that he go for some testing brought to me a sense of relief. Finally we would have some answers to this thing, whatever it was, that was impairing this man of mine, and that had been niggling at the back of my mind for these several years.

Watching Dave pick up twigs was only the introduction to a new and cruel reality.

Gwen Bibber Kimball

Chapter 2

DENIAL

As I share some of the personal details of our lives it is done with the hope that perhaps the relating of them might provide encouragement to others who find themselves groping in darkness and confusion, totally unaware of the reason for it all.

I found myself increasingly mystified during those early days as we unknowingly approached the great valley which was lying directly ahead of David Kimball. It was to present totally unfamiliar ground to both of us. Handling events after enlightenment is quite different from wandering around, hit and miss, in the obscure surroundings which characterize early days of wondering and questioning.

Prior to the twig days, back in the '80's somewhere, I had begun encountering a recurring and mystifying response from Dave, "I didn't know that." It was mystifying because the subject was not new to him, and I knew Dave did "know that". It was said in several different ways. Sometimes it was "I never heard that before;" sometimes "I never knew that," or "I knew nothing about that;" sometimes "You never told me that." These responses started slowly, and became more and more intrusive in our attempts to communicate.

Dave's not understanding or answering simple questions; his saying over and over, "You weren't clear," even after I struggled to rephrase sentences into first grade vocabulary; his short-term memory loss; his breaking into the middle of a simple discussion by saying, "I don't know what you're talking about," (which caused me to feel a wave of nausea the first time I encountered it); these incidents increased my consternation. I also became aware of Dave's watching television more and more, and with what seemed like undue and mindless attention to even the ads. Those, and other events, were increasingly alarming to me.

When you know otherwise, what do you do with these events as they first enter your life? I found myself to be at a total loss. I was perplexed; I was even somewhat annoyed; I was suspicious. Of what? I was not sure.

The human mind, mine at least, does all sorts of gymnastics as it tries to deal with events which deny reality. Something here was not making any sense. My mind told me that much, although not much more.

As time passed I tried to rationalize what Dave's motive could be in denying what I knew to be true, and what he also should know to be true. I had no way of knowing that he no longer knew what was true. Considerable time was to elapse before I would understand this.

I had never been the kind of wife who made secret plans and then surprised her husband with them, but for some reason that was exactly what Dave seemed to be thinking. No amount of reviewing and reassuring made any difference. His response usually was, "You're mistaken," always stated with authority and finality. I was to find out, eventually, that he was increasingly unable to remember much of what he had recently heard. Short-term memory loss. I did not know about that yet.

I recall, in the early '90's, the evening we were expected to attend a dine-out dinner, an occasion where each assigned couple provided an agreed-upon portion of the meal. It might be a casserole, a vegetable dish or whatever. Because of the nature of the dinner it was important that each guest take seriously the responsibility for attending.

The event was talked about at home during the day of the dinner, and I prepared my dish for the meal. About an hour before departure time I reminded Dave so that he could be ready. He announced that he knew nothing of this dinner and furthermore he didn't feel like going. I was flabbergasted!

He steadfastly denied having been consulted about any such dinner or of having agreed to go. No amount of discussion changed his mind, not even the issue of our obligation toward the hostess. This was one of the first evidences that attempts at reasoning were to become futile. I did not know about that yet, either.

A dinner for eight was obviously going to be a dinner for seven, and I could go alone. His casual attitude about my having to find my way, after dark, to an area with which I was totally unfamiliar left my emotions in a tail-spin, and there were those mild ill thoughts again.

Another occasion was the evening of one of our wedding anniversaries. Dave, in spite of my attempts to change his mind, chose to stay home and work on a project while I went by myself with friends for a social evening. My mentality shook its head in disbelief. More perplexity. More ill thoughts.

But this was not Dave Kimball. If not he, then who was it? Who was this person I was beginning not to know: self-centered, incapable of reason, wary, remote?

At first I would firmly press the point that he indeed had been told of plans, that he did once know and had apparently just forgotten. That approach generated more heat than light. Dave was sure that his memory, which had been one of his fortes, could not possibly be the problem. And indeed he had had a phenomenal memory, as was attested to by his college days. I remembered drilling him on his definitions for a course in Abnormal Psychology and had marveled at a mind that could retain so much intricate material and quote it so flawlessly and rapidly.

I backed away from that approach until finally it became apparent even to Dave himself that he certainly was forgetting things. For instance, time after time upon his returning from the grocery store with an odd assortment of things, he would find his list in his pocket, forgotten, no memory of my having given it to him. Yet, here was the mute evidence that I had done so. That issue, perhaps more than anything else, stimulated reality thinking for Dave.

Eventually, after events like this became routine, emotions and reality collided. I was no longer alone in the realization that we obviously had a problem of considerable proportion, the source of which we as yet did not know. At this point, depression descended on Dave like a cloud.

Increasingly I became accustomed to the possibility of changing plans the last minute, of being constantly on the alert to just hang loose and let what was going to happen, happen. That course of action made it easier for both of us, perhaps most of all for me. I learned to entertain no expectations. I settled into a routine of adjusting, sometimes graciously, sometimes ungraciously, all the while becoming increasingly troubled.

These were bewildering days. They evidenced an era of crisis in the life of Dave Kimball that was typical of a specific illness which I cared not to even consider, and about which we knew little, but about which we were destined to learn a great deal more. Until we did learn just what that specific illness was, the intervening interlude was a study in frustration and perplexity, as is the case for all those who are destined to walk this path.

Our daughter Karen, when learning to put words together as a child, had a cute little way of expressing something she didn't know about by saying, "I can't know that." In her little-girl way she was expressing not only what her Dad was saying, but what was now going on with our family. Something destined to be long-termed and destructive was reaching into our lives. We couldn't know that.

Chapter 3

REALITY

Shortly after Dave's recovery from his neck fracture he underwent a series of tests and x-rays in an attempt to determine the cause or causes of his distressing situation. No physical basis was detected, though there was agreement on the presence of memory loss, and of some ability to reason, along with the obvious depression.

After a trial period on several medications with no positive results, Dr. Michael Fiori, Psychiatrist, entered our lives in 1996. His presence brought enormous comfort and support. We met with him regularly, giving him the opportunity to assess Dave's state. During these months the mystery deepened and I could feel only profound gratitude that there was now a kind, caring professional in our lives to help us find our way through what had become, to me, a classic maze.

After Dr. Fiori had met with us for some months he urged me to call him at any time if I had questions, or felt a need to talk with him. Eventually, upon returning home from an appointment I did just that. Having become aware of the symptoms of one specific illness I felt compelled to ask him in private, "Are we dealing with Alzheimer's here?" His answer? "OH YES."

The question I had tried to tuck away finally had an answer. The gray area of sky cleared somewhat. I can't say it caused the sun to shine brightly, but at least we could now discern our landscape. That discerning brought with it a mixture of emotions, one of which was relief, another dismay: relief because we now knew where we were, and we now knew our enemy; dismay because by now I was at least partially cognizant of the implications of that diagnosis, and had some idea where it could eventually take us. We would find out soon enough where we were going.

There is no point in looking back. We are living in the now. But I do realize that on many occasions my understanding would have been greater, and my approach different, had I realized just what was beginning to take place in our lives. We could have avoided some tense and unhappy situations, had we only known.

There is also no point in looking ahead. God's Word tells us, and good judgment and just plain old common sense concur, that we deal with one day at a time, and indeed that is all that we can handle. Time will surely bear that out.

Alzheimer's is today a household word and everyone is in a more knowledgeable position to bring aid and comfort to both the afflicted and the caregiver. My encouragement, even exhortation, to others who have suspicions that something is not right with a loved one, is to seek counsel, aggressively and early. One of you needs to understand what is going on.

Finally I understood, and with the impact of that understanding all things changed. Nothing helps a difficult situation like knowing that you have one on your hands. From that point on you can start making the necessary, even compelling, adjustments toward a future that is sensitive to the needs that will exist in both lives.

Without delay, Dave and I sat down together at my request. I held his hand in mine, and I told him, as gently as I knew how, what I had just learned from Dr. Fiori. How did Dave accept the diagnosis? Mercifully for both of us, he had almost no memory of ever having heard the word, "Alzheimer's." His response was the rather bland comment, "Well, at least what is wrong with me has a name."

He did, however, begin to ask about symptoms, causes, the future, etc. He seemed to feel not only comforted, but relieved, to do so, which led us to many times of talking quietly together. He would soon forget that we had already talked, so we went over the same ground often, as if it were the first time around.

Periodically, although not as often as at the onset, he still asks the same questions, and seems satisfied, temporarily -- until he forgets the details again. However, though the details quickly disappear from his mind, he is ever aware of the fact of his impairment. His most fervent hope is that I will be here with him as he walks this walk, though he does not really realize from day to day where that walk could and may take him. Again, mercifully for both of us.

One of our first steps into the future was a decision that we, together, would tell anyone with whom we had any intimate contact, that Dave indeed has Alzheimer's. This was one of our wisest decisions. It allows people to understand his memory and reasoning losses, and Dave is no longer on guard as he would have been had we been trying to keep a secret. It gives others the liberty to reveal the presence of an illness of their own. It becomes a meeting place where mutual honesty provides comfort and support for each heart.

Just a few days after the decision to let people know, we had occasion to enjoy lunch with two old friends. Dave immediately told Stan, "Well, I've just been diagnosed with

Alzheimer's." Stan replied, "Good for you for being open about it, Dave. Now I can tell you that I've just been diagnosed with Parkinson's." They felt totally free to share thoughts about their plights. I'm sure it brought a measure of comfort to both. My reaction was, "How wonderful not to be hiding."

I would strongly advise couples and families to be openly "up front". Even the people at the market need to understand why Dave is apt to load groceries into the cart without having the cashier place them into a bag first. Everyone relaxes when I say, "My husband has Alzheimer's and sometimes forgets the need for bags." I have never sensed the slightest embarrassment.

Dr. Fiori is very present in our lives these days and is one of our wonderful support people. I thank him over and over for "being there." I doubt that he has any idea how important his presence is to the Kimballs, and especially to me. I can call him at any time for opinions or advice, for a medication adjustment, or if only to inform him of any change in Dave's condition. These all help us find our way more easily, and in my world that makes him a mainstay.

I no longer cry when I observe Dave picking up twigs. It is kind that we can become accustomed to change. As a couple our individual needs are now different, because one member of this union is moving into a mysterious state of confusion, depression, and isolation. That means that I also have, out ahead of me, a slowly but surely and constantly changing mode of life to which I must learn to adjust. Alzheimer's is to become a heartless and persistent saboteur of our journey together.

Chapter 4

NON-TRUST

What impact does this relentless intruder called Alzheimer's make upon the innate personality of its victim? What added stresses are placed upon who that person really is?

As I ponder these questions and try to analyze them as they relate to this Kimball family, I need to go back many years and refer to a basic struggle in Dave's life -- that of difficulty in trusting people.

The struggle arose during childhood, due mainly to his emotional response to a grandmother who lived in the home, and who thought his older brother should have been the only grandchild in the family. She left no doubt as to her attitude, and unfortunately the feelings that were generated in the small child's mind prevailed into adulthood. He passed those feelings off for years by referring to his grandmother as "a demon on little red wheels," always said in a jocular manner, followed by a big hearty laugh -- the ultimate in cover-ups.

His brother Bob, at the same time, felt that his parents favored David, the natural result, I assume, of their trying to compensate for the attitude of Grandmother, without open confrontation. Everyone suffered. Forthrightness would have been better.

Dave says he learned by age five that no one would defend him against her. That message caused him to "know what he knew -- he didn't really matter that much." Consequently, who could you trust? Surely not anyone close to you. His dearest ally was his cousin Frances, who was like a sister to him, but to whom he never revealed his distress.

Grandmother had already imposed her substantial matriarchal propensities upon her own three children, one of whom was Dave's mother. None had been allowed to finish high school. Grandfather covered his clandestine visits with his married children as "taking a walk." All had found it prudent, apparently, to choose compliance in lieu of defiance. Unfortunately it seems that in some cases the matriarchs of society and family are not to be challenged. Obviously, such was the mind-set there.

I came into the family when Dave was pursuing his formal education during his early to mid twenties. Grandmother still lived in the home, and that attitude toward him was still very apparent to me. He continued to be an emotional victim to this subject at times, even into his 80's.

His mother once told me that she had found it hard to cross her mother; she "didn't want to have any regrets." I asked her if she had any about permitting Gram's treatment of her son and she said, "Yes."

Dave's parents were good, sincere, hardworking people who lived a very provincial, subjugated life. To them, responsibility to one's family was mainly a matter of providing the essentials for daily living, and teaching spiritual and moral values. Those things were done diligently. I have no doubt they loved their children deeply.

However, there was little of any personal relationship among family members. Physical contact was almost nonexistent, and hugs from me, after I entered the family produced blushing and embarrassment. I remember Dave's mother stating to me that she felt it was possible to love someone without having to show it. My response, as a non-subtle 20-year-old, "Why in the world would anyone want to do that?" was probably not the ultimate in diplomacy, but a philosophy of that sort was unthinkable to me.

Indeed, teaching Dave Kimball how to receive and show love has been one of my challenges during our years together, and showing him love in his present circumstance is one of our family's most important functions.

I am sure, in their emotionally inhibited way, his parents were proud of him, but they seemed unaware of the need to show him their overt support and approval. They were not present when he was the Valedictorian speaker at his college commencement. They chose to be absent on the day of his wedding (which was in another state), mourning instead the death of Grandmother whom, they commented, "had seemed to plan even her death to hurt David."

They were, without doubt, products of their own backgrounds as we all are. Probably they would have handled parenting differently if they could have been the recipients of some of the valuable insights such as those found today in ministries of people like Dr. James Dobson who so skillfully focuses on the family. Who of us wouldn't do some things differently if we could go back to our parenting days? But certain emotions were in place for Dave, and those emotions set him up for non-trust. "I felt deserted back there," Dave says.

Long before he was aware, on the conscious level, that such a problem of non-trust existed, those of us within the family who knew him on a day-to-day basis in adulthood, picked up symptoms over and over again. They mainly expressed an inability to let people get close to him, both physically and emotionally. That restraint extended itself not only to the general public, but especially to the immediate family. The guard was always up and in place to varying degrees.

But he interfaced this struggle with growing up, marrying, becoming a dad, attaining top status in college, and fulfilling a fruitful pastoral ministry of thirty years duration. To those thirty years add the founding of a chaplain ministry known as the Community Chaplain Service, a one-on-one ministry to the elderly in nursing homes, and you have a picture of a very bright and capable man who achieved much.

During those years he seemed to be unaware of his feelings of non-trust, and he used his fine mind mainly as a sharply-honed teaching tool. It in fact became his chief ally. He was convinced of the need for people to know what God's Word really was saying, and he reveled in making Biblical doctrine relevant to, and clearly understood by, those who sat under his ministry.

After acquiring his own family the long-buried subject of non-trust surfaced. But it would not be until our daughters were in their teens that finally we were able to talk openly and honestly, about his complicated array of emotions. Among these feelings was a deep-seated anger which he had not admitted even to himself, and which he had managed to keep quite well hidden.

His admission to the presence of this anger was probably the beginning of the healing process. After many years of reflection Dave decided that Grandmother must have had her own baggage which made her who she was. He also came to realize that she, as well as his parents, were indeed debtors to him, which debt he finally became willing and able to forgive, at least intellectually. The emotional part of that forgiveness is still a struggle which surfaces easily. As with most injuries, the scars remain. Dealing with the effects of Alzheimer's does not facilitate that process.

As I look back at Dave's years of feeling deserted and angry, I believe those feelings became the catalyst for his burden for the nursing home residents. He was able to connect with those who were also feeling deserted and angry. What a lovely picture of an omnipotent God turning a hurt into a ministry.

However, as Dave finds he can no longer depend upon that which was once his chief ally, his intellect, he is being forced more and more into dependency upon those of us at home, entrusting to us nearly every detail of his life, even in areas that are normally most private. He often states that he feels he is back living in Grandmother's world. Someone is always checking on where he is and what he is doing, just as in his little boy days. At that point he often loses sight of our love and loyalty, and his fragile trust vanishes.

His reactions are those of frustration and at times, anger -- anger over his situation, and anger at us for our invasions. We, as his support family, try to eliminate as many situations as we can that would cause him to be aware of his need to trust us. But even with our caution, and even though he realizes that he is laboring under waning mental powers, it must be devastating to him when he senses our intrusions. Sometimes he explodes when we have to interfere, and says things like, "Anyone would think I can't do anything by myself." Tragically, that pretty much states it, but how eroding that fact must be to whatever remains of his ego and self-esteem, especially when trust is such an issue.

At times, he expresses momentary anger at God for allowing him to be in this situation. We allow him to vent without rebuke. He does not need guilt added to the reality that trust for him is no longer an option. It has become an odious and scary imperative.

It is especially critical that I, as the primary caregiver, stay aware of my role which at times becomes a tightrope. I realize, at those times, how easy it would be for me to further victimize Dave by causing issues, or even by pointing them out, unless it is absolutely necessary to do so. It is critical that I try to balance his mental loss with his feelings, and that I keep in mind where he is having to walk. I don't always accomplish this.

It is also critical that he feel the overt support and approval of his entire family at this time in his life. I surmise that we all learn rather slowly about this illness and its inroads into a life. Because of its elusiveness, understanding may dawn on us late, but we can make sure now that it is not too little.

We conclude that for David Kimball, this relentless intruder is a demon with two programs. One robs him of his most precious mental faculties, and the other demands that he trust, in the face of that loss -- an almost impossible assignment for him. His mental faculties were his life. Trust was always fleeting.

However, it does seem that he is gaining some confidence in us, perhaps because we are coping better and he is feeling more comfortable with that. Increasingly he seems to depend on our being here for him. How rewarding for us.

Alzheimer's is indeed an evil, not only in our lives, but in the lives of all who encounter its cruel and devastating consequences. Who we are, what scars we carry, what painful areas of our lives are to be further exposed, those and other components will impact the lives of entire families, both victims and caregivers. Each will need to find ways to deal with his own particular involvements in the midst of this struggle.

Gwen Bibber Kimball

Chapter 5

SELF-ESTEEM

No matter how we are put together emotionally, one of the most important factors for successful living is how we regard ourselves as we attempt to live useful and productive lives. In this area the Alzheimer's victim suffers one of his most painful and degrading blows because Alzheimer's is a degrading illness. This is especially true when one's vocation has been specifically dependent upon a well-oiled and smoothly running mind, which now runs by fits and starts, certainly not smoothly.

With the mental losses which are so rapidly changing who he has always been, I ponder how much there is left for Dave Kimball's inner person to feel good about. He grew up with somewhat meager feelings of self-worth. College became a place where he could look at himself differently, and his personhood took on legitimacy. He says of those days, "I found my safe place in academics. They rescued me from my feelings of worthlessness. I was finally attaining. I could feel good about myself. Classmates kidded me about my grades and I guess that gave me a boost."

I remember how proud I was of him when he was inducted into the Gordon College Honor Society, "Phi Alpha Chi," in 1946, an honor he had earned by diligent attention to his studies, at the same time functioning as a husband, a father, and a student pastor. However, he appeared to pass completely over this honor; he has never attended an Honor Society meeting and has no idea where his key is. If it were I, I would have it hanging around my neck, dangling from my ear or a charm bracelet, or at least in some very obvious place, with appropriate humility, of course! The sad part is, I can't even find it.

Any attempt over the years to encourage him to become a part of the Society has been met with disdain. I can only conclude that even with this high honor, the old feelings of non-worth plugged in, and he was not able to regard himself highly enough to enjoy participation.

Now, due to Alzheimer's, the thrust of those days is past and he is experiencing a bereavement over his waning intellect as real as if he were grieving the loss of a loved one. Most of his very fragile self-esteem has gone away to some mysterious, strangely out-of-touch place. He says he feels only partially connected to the person he once knew.

Even his connection to God becomes vague at times and he feels he is, for all practical purposes, a relatively unimportant member of society, now that he is so mentally handicapped.

He used to say quite often, at the onset of this illness, "I used to have a brain." I could feel only anguish and anger over anything that could so reduce his self-esteem.

One of the by-products of Dave's reliance upon his former mental capabilities was a feeling, among those of us who comprise his immediate family, that we were not especially needed in order for him to fulfill who and what he was. His isolation into his own brand of mental and emotional self-sufficiency allowed him to exist adequately, for him, in a rather distant and private place with his books. Living in solitude was simply doing what he had learned to do during boyhood.

When I found I must adjust to that remoteness I was mystified and thoroughly shaken. I couldn't imagine life in such an impersonal climate. I struggled for months, all the while loving him but feeling as if I couldn't find him. One morning I read in the Book of Joshua what was to become a prophecy in my life: "In three days you shall pass over this Jordan ... be strong and courageous." I knew that on the other side of the Jordan River lay Canaan, the land of promise and of milk and honey. After deep pondering, and fervent prayer, I dared myself to take that promise as my own. When I did, God provided a miracle -- that of an accepting and challenged heart. On that day I got on with my life. I remember it vividly.

Unfortunately I was too young and inexperienced to realize the impact that Dave's remoteness would have on our children. In adulthood both Midge and Karen share the opinion that they never really knew their Dad back there. How sad for both father and children. My question to myself will always be, "Could I have done more?"

As I witness his new level of aloneness brought on by Alzheimer's, I constantly search in my mind for some way to offset this awful circumstance he finds himself in. How could we as a family prevent this somewhat guarded man from withdrawing further into himself?

Reason tells me that Dave now has a great need to know of the esteem, the respect, the love, and the approval that we as a family, along with his multitude of friends, feel for him. Reason also tells me that we now have a marvelous opportunity to support him and help fill the void in his life in ways that we've never been able to do before. With his one important ally disappearing, he is not only very vulnerable. He is in a position to be very receptive. Karen expressed something we are all feeling: "We now know we are needed." How liberating and challenging that fact is for everyone involved.

One morning as we sat and visited warmly together, we wondered how many families in this day are able to do what we were doing. The girls and I have done this often, and now we feel that even though our Dad is limited, he has become part of the family in a new way. He is most eager to hear our comments and to know the subjects of our conversations. It appears that this is an almost frantic attempt on his part to stay in touch. We continue to help him do that, even though subjects and their meanings are very likely to drop quickly out of sight. His progressive hearing loss further complicates matters.

He still surprises us occasionally by coming up with great one-liners. One night recently our supper was delayed substantially from its quite regular 5:45 hour. After waiting for some time and seeing no prospects of eating right away (a casserole was out of sight in the oven), Dave strolled out where I was and said, "Well, what's for breakfast?" That was a flash of the old David, and of course my applause was immediate, and his smile was smug.

While it is sad that sometimes it takes bad things to help us refocus, it is also gratifying that good things can result. Dave discusses his old remote feelings with openness now, whenever his head is working. "I regret the former order of things in life," he stated recently, "ministry first, then family. That was not only the spiritual order in those days, it was also where I was most comfortable, but certainly it was the wrong order. Now I can understand why my girls did not really get to know their Dad."

For all that Alzheimer's has taken out of Dave's life, we have received in return an avenue of communication which was unexpected, and is infinitely valued.

The challenge for us, his family, is to find every way possible to let this man of worth know that he is just that -- a man of worth. Mental excellence doesn't matter. He matters. Our hope is that in our attempting to carry out this challenge, something vital and fulfilling will flood his consciousness and satisfy the void that is being created, as his mind continues to fail him.

We are attempting to erase his feelings of remoteness by expressing more warmth, more encouragement, more approval, more hugs -- all those good things. Our message to him is one of appreciation for who he is, without fostering any erroneous thought on his part that this is just a palliative and pacifying program we have set ourselves on. That would be patronage.

As is always the case, those who are now giving of themselves in this variety of ways are receiving a greater blessing than they are giving. Isn't that what the promise was all about? "Give, and it shall be given unto you ... For with the same measure that ye measure it shall be measured to you again." Luke 6:38 (KJV)

As the mother, I feel great joy in observing Dave's daughters expressing their concerns for their father's plight. It is also heartening for me to observe the pleasure he derives from every bit of bolstering he receives. To the best of our human ability we are committed daily to protecting whatever measure of self-esteem he has, for whatever aware-time he has left.

Gwen Bibber Kimball

Chapter 6

PLATEAUS

As a native-born New Englander I am accustomed to both ocean and hills, and I notice immediately any change from that type of geographical environment. After choosing early on in his ministry to move to the Midwest to pursue further education, Dave went on ahead, in 1948, to prepare for us to join him there. Some weeks later I left on the train from South Station in Boston with our two daughters, Midge, age 4, and Karen, 3 months, in a compartment on the New England Wolverine. In the waning daylight I enjoyed observing the lovely Berkshires, not aware of the changes that would take place in the landscape while we slept and the train made its way west.

Incidents during the night caused me to wonder. At one point we were awakened by jostling and shunting of cars from track to track. Also, we seemed not to be following the route laid out in our time schedule. I paid scant attention, and felt no special concern. The powers that be surely knew what they were about.

Upon awaking in the morning in Indiana and raising the curtain on our window I did not have to be too perceptive a person to realize the vast changes I was gazing out upon. I will never forget the shock I felt. While we were not looking, things had changed. It was as if, during that long night, we had been transported to another planet. First, no trees. Second, I could see forever. All of a sudden my world was starkly different. Outside that window my new world appeared to be one huge plateau.

The land was so flat that all roads came to a point on the horizon. They were lined on both sides by huge fields of green corn. Trees, when there were any, were younger and smaller than those to which we were accustomed. Soil was black and rich, and unlike New England, there were no stones.

These and other details took some getting used to but eventually, after several years at our destination in Illinois, we did begin to see the beauty in the fields of corn that seemed to wave forever in the almost constant breeze which blew across the prairies. We took great comfort in getting to Lake Michigan as often as possible. The fragrance was somewhat different but we were delighted to find seagulls. The magnificent surf at the southern end of the lake almost made us forget we were not at the ocean.

Nothing could ever compete with our hills and ocean, in my humble although probably prejudiced opinion, but wonderful people helped fill the gap, and we adjusted gradually to our new geography and found happiness there for over 12 years.

As I remember the changes we were thrust into at the time, I compare them with the changes which had taken place in our lives when, in 1996, we pushed up the curtain on a landscape known as Alzheimer's. Again, one did not have to be too perceptive to recognize that our world was quite a different one. There had been those unsettling events during another long night that lay behind us, and we had wondered at our unfamiliar, and certainly unscheduled route. But again, we had trusted the Powers that be to get us where we were supposed to be, and again, while we were not looking, things had indeed changed.

It seemed that our landscape consisted of a succession of ever-changing plateaus, one after another, each requiring its own adjustment as Dave progressively exhibited the inability to remember, to reason, or to understand simple thoughts. I had always thought of looking up at plateaus, each one slightly higher than the last. Suddenly I found that this new landscape presented the opposite view. Each of our new plateaus was requiring a look downward, because that is the only direction an Alzheimer's patient can go.

According to the dictionary a plateau is a table-like surface, deeply cut by valleys of various depths and widths. That definition quite aptly depicts the landscape of those who deal with this illness, both victim and caregiver. Life becomes a combination of fairly smooth, navigable areas, interrupted by sometimes gentle, sometimes rough crossings over shallow or deep streams, all of which eventually level off onto that next lower plateau.

One continually wanders around these areas, wondering just where they will eventually take you. Sometime in the future I assume one of them could be the step into that great valley of total non-comprehension. For myself, I dread the probability of having to view that plateau, but at times I find myself welcoming it for Dave. It will diminish his painful awareness, even though it will add immensely to the level of his care.

Surprises become less surprising, and unpredictable behavior is more commonplace as the landscape increasingly becomes something neither of us recognizes. Valleys appear more often, frequently taking on the depth of gorges, and the smooth places appear less frequently. Unlike our experience in the Midwest, we do not have time to adjust to all the changes as they occur here.

I acquiesce to the fact of our changed landscape, realizing at the same time how much I have to learn from it. We both are encouraged by our supportive family, our close friends, and by our willingness to readjust our sights to our new horizons. But mostly, our daily, even momentary reliance upon our God is our pillar.

For Dave Kimball, who has led a busy life, time seems to go on endlessly, and it has become his one big enemy as he drops from plateau to plateau. He is basically not a hobby man. But if you walked into his room or the family room and observed the area around his chair you would suspect that he has a love affair with books. They are everywhere. A few days ago I gathered up 11 from around one chair and shortly they had been replaced by three more.

But I am noticing a change of plateau even in this, his great love. Reading for understanding and enlightenment is slowly giving place to disjointed attempts at reading scattered portions of several books, going from one to another as if he were just nibbling away at a meal: a little potato, a taste of dessert, a bite of chicken, some coffee... I doubt that there is any continuity of thought, but at least he is doing that which is so dear to him -- spending time with good books. Thankfully it does help him pass some of those endless hours.

Before the diagnosis of Alzheimer's, while Dave was still able to function fairly adequately, he had what he called a Resource Center at Mullein Hill Church: a wide selection of books on display on Sunday mornings, to be loaned out as in a Library. Giving this ministry up was one of his early steps downward. I deeply regretted the time when he no longer felt able to carry on. It had been good for him, and it had encouraged many people to pursue that which has become almost a lost art, the art of reading.

Just now he is attempting to read our story about the Community Chaplain Service, "You Say WHAT, Lord?", and he has no memory of having read it several times, or of even having seen it before. Whether or not he understands or remembers anything he reads is of little concern to me now. Please God, may he not soon become disinterested in this one diversion which has been the love of his life.

With the passing of time, new plateaus continue to appear. Dave loved to tinker in the garage with his tools. He could always find something to saw, split or nail. The awareness of his real illness caused many changes. Dr. Fiori took full responsibility for eliminating his Skil-saw from his life. He missed it and asked about it over and over for months, and as has been our practice, I told him each time, honestly, that his Doctor felt he should no longer risk using it. Dave didn't understand why that was necessary, but he complied, perhaps mainly out of respect and love for Dr. Fiori. Thankfully, he finally forgot it. Along the way we had to eliminate the power lawnmower, weed trimmer, and leaf-eater. He finally forgot those also, and eventually he even forgot Dr. Fiori.

Another plateau that continually constricts his life is that of a much smaller social world. His memory of family and friends is shrinking almost daily, unless he has consistent visual contact with them. The girls planned a week of R and R for me one year -- Karen took me to Niagara Falls. Midgie came and stayed with her Dad. He could not remember her, and in spite of much explaining he apparently felt he had been left with a stranger. One day while Midgie had him out for a ride Dave said, "We're having such a good conversation -- it would be nice to know who you are." Midgie replied, "I'm your kid, Dad, I'm Midgie." "Oh," responded her Dad, "I wish Gwen were here. I'd like for her to meet you."

When in public it seems that he guards his mental losses by appearing to be a stand-up comic, which he has never been, though he has always had a good sense of humor and has been an inveterate pun artist. Now he seems to feel the need to have a humorous quip as a response to anyone who approaches him. His uneasy groping for words becomes obvious. This in itself puts pressure on him, if I am reading correctly the expression in his eyes and his too-hearty smile.

But at times his quips are good ones. One day he was trying to converse with a lady at church and, of course, forgot his train of thought. She graciously said, "Never mind, Dave. When you get to Heaven you won't have any of these things to worry about." "Oh yes," he said, "I'll still have one worry." "What is that?", she asked. Dave jerked his thumb in my direction and said, "If she doesn't get there who will make my coffee?"

The possibility of an in-depth conversation absolutely terrifies him. I try to stand in the gap and rescue him when it appears he is not able to handle things by himself and he stays very close by, when we are in public. He prefers to go to the safety of the car which now is always kept locked, of course, and I dare not leave him with the keys. Another plateau, and another humiliation for him.

He has been able to handle praying aloud at home quite well until recently. He now occasionally loses his way and has to be helped to finish. I notice increasingly that his prayers are more a matter of rote, and he is apt to forget what he desires to pray about. Sadly his prayer world is getting smaller. Another plateau.

One is easily lulled into a placid state during the course of this illness. It is easy to feel that you have found your pace with each new change. Not true. One morning recently Dave got up not knowing whether it was morning, afternoon, or evening, except that the sun was shining in a certain window which caused him to assume that it was morning. "Besides," he said, "I just got up so it must be morning, and my watch says 6:45 and that must be 6:45 am . . . " Even after my confirming that it was indeed morning, we had to go over it all again and again in order for him to be sure.

This was a first, and I found that at this point I dropped to a new plateau with him, and was reminded again that nothing is stable here. That's the rule. I keep thinking I know that, but my occasional feelings of mild surprise tell me it is easy to be off guard. Probably just about the time I've become accustomed to things as they are, the plateau will change. This must be a perfect example of on-the-job training.

I cannot even imagine what our next plateaus will be, but as I anticipate them I pray they will not yet be too unkind. Time will tell. Whatever they are we shall bathe them in prayer, and attempt to handle them appropriately. As my heart sings along with a Gaither video these days I very often ask myself what in the world I would ever do "If the Lord wasn't walking by my side."

Chapter 7

EARLY ENIGMAS

As people ask me, "When were you first aware that something was wrong?", I take a long look at the years that lie behind us. I find myself remembering events from a Monday-morning-quarterbacking perspective. From this vantage point certain events still stand out conspicuously. They stood out back there, but I didn't know why.

Those were the years when we were involved with our pastorates. Some of those churches had very special groups of Young People and many of our best years of ministry were spent with them. It seemed our house was always full. Sometimes it was a pizza party. Often it was sitting by the fireplace after church on Sunday evening with Cokes and "S'mores." Sometimes they just dropped in for a visit on their way home from school.

In winter you might find them with a toboggan on the hill behind our house, with styrofoam cups of hot chocolate parked on a snow bank, a heavy rope laced between trees to help pull themselves back up the steep slope from the ice-covered lake.

One year we took a group to Mad River in New Hampshire's White Mountains for a weekend of camping -- a tent for girls -- a tent for boys. As someone has said, "There wasn't a single mosquito there; they were all married and had huge families." Indeed, they were there by the millions, and all the bug spray would have been gone the first night except that we herded the kids into their tents at bedtime with a final spraying and then confiscated the cans for the next day. I can still remember that tent full of giggly girls all snuggled down in their sleeping bags, as we said final prayers, did that final spraying for the night, and then zipped up the flap.

We rescued dental retainers (safely wrapped in a napkin?) from the campfire, we climbed Mr. Osceola with our peanut butter sandwiches, candy bars and bottles of soda; we had a church service sitting on the rocks in the sunshine by the riverbed on Sunday morning, followed by a challenging swim in the frigid water. We've kept all those pictures as some of our treasures.

One Saturday we took them on a "hobo" breakfast. They each had their own stoves made from large-sized cans, open end down, windows cut in the side through which to feed their fires. They had three matches each. They gathered wood for their own fires, cooked their bacon on the tops of their cans, and then pinched their eggs open to fry in the bacon fat. We did take extra eggs, fortunately, because it became obvious that some of those youngsters had never cracked an egg open before that morning. Theirs missed the cans and landed with a plop into the dirt. Last of all, the batter for a pancake was poured onto the top of each can. Parts of it were hilarious, and even though it was a damp, foggy morning no one seemed to notice.

These young people were some of our very special human beings and we loved being with them. We spent hours talking with them, teaching them, and praying with them. I could not have imagined a time when they would not be a large part of our lives.

But, as happens in the Ministry, the pastor moves on to another church and you live through the teary farewells with your special ones, and carry your memories with you for many years.

Upon our return to their area somewhere in the 70's a group of these same young people, now grown up, some married, asked their once Pastor K. to have a Bible study for them. I was ecstatic. He refused them. I was stunned. It was so out of character for him to respond to them in that manner.

I pleaded, and probably got an attitude over it, all to no avail. No reasoning of mine could change his mind. I asked a simple "Why?" No answer. Dave absolutely refused to discuss it.

From this present vantage point I can now view one of our early plateaus. At that time it was as yet unidentifiable. I pondered for years, never quite understanding what had changed.

However, I had begun to notice back there that when asked a specific question, Dave would often ignore it and answer something else. I wondered why he did that. Was he not recognizing the actual question (hardly likely, it seemed), or was he no longer able to come up with the answer on the spot?

We talked about that, or rather I did. I suggested, if that were a problem for him, that he just say something such as, "That's a good question. Let's write it down and work it out next time." That would take the pressure off and give him time to think. And as I further reminded him, no one has all the answers at his fingertips, no matter how bright he is. My conversation about it remained a monologue. Again, Dave refused to discuss it. It was as if he was confronted with a huge mental roadblock. Apparently he was. "We couldn't know that." These, and many other issues continued to add to my consternation.

I finally concluded that he feared being put on the spot with questions; he was able to preach a good sermon, but that was monologue, with no intervals allowing for input that he might not be able to handle.

That event stands out as one of my first mysteries which remained unsolved for many years, until we finally met our enemy 20 years later. Then I understood.

As I go back over those years I recall more and more events that were mysteries to me: Dave's disregarding of the rules of the highway; the many dents and dings I kept finding on the car; his complete lack of memory for oil changes; forgetting to pay bills on time, etc. These things seemed to me to imply carelessness and inattention. Not knowing then that it was the beginning of an illness, I pondered.

So we moved into that long night of increasingly unpredictable behavior. Dave was oblivious. I alone sensed that our lives were reaching a confusing turning point. And as I write this I wonder how many others out there are struggling over the same sorts of issues, and are also pondering and agonizing, as I did.

Chapter 8

DEATH OF A MIND

I am reminded of the comments of a friend who has been in my life for some years. She shared with me how desperately hard it was to lose her husband as quickly as she had lost hers. She felt she had insufficient time to prepare, and because he did not talk easily about things like death, they had no opportunity to grieve together. She longed to hold him and cry with him over the shortening of their years together. She wanted to talk of Heaven. None of that happened, and her grief feels unfinished.

As I compare grief with grief, I observe my own. I am experiencing not the death of a man, but the death of a man's mind. That death marches relentlessly on, and on, and on, and is a grief comparable to, even exceeding, a physical death, in my estimation. It is neither painfully quick, nor shockingly over as my friend's experience was. It is at first tantalizingly elusive, and then it is painfully slow, and shockingly expansive. It asserts itself into every phase of life. The forgetfulness, mental confusion, and accompanying frustration, anger and depression become an agony for both of us, and cause me to yearn for Heaven for this one who has become the victim, and who is now so very aware, yet so very unaware, of his limitations.

Dave takes a deep breath. "I am so glad I am no longer responsible for the Church or the Chaplain work," he says. Shortly the tears come. "But I will never preach again, or visit with my Chaplains again," he continues, as he gives vent to his sorrow and bereavement.

The struggle is so sad. How to comfort? No sermonette is appropriate here. Words are not only inadequate. They seem trite and banal.

As I witness the struggle, one of the most effective supports I am able to give is to "commune", a word with a very special meaning to those in our household. It is a sort of love-in between two people, a time of holding and stroking, cheek against cheek, warm, close and quiet. Sometimes it is a brief encounter. At other times it is more prolonged, and often there is a reluctance to terminate the melding of two human spirits who, for the moment, know they are being understood and supported by each other. This sort of contact was not common during Dave's growing up days, but I can tell by his reluctance at times to "let go" that he feels comforted and senses love.

And then there are the occasions where any such encounter is flatly refused. "You're smothering me," he says. So be it. We go on to other things.

Some years ago Dave started shutting his eyes when he was feeling confused, or when his ability to reason appeared to be inadequate. That tendency has increased. It seems that by so doing he is indicating his overwhelming feelings of helplessness, and is closing not just his eyes, but also his mind to that which has become unbearable. I assume that this is a defense mechanism, and probably is a necessary one, in his attempt to shut out that which he can no longer handle. At this point I doubt that he even hears. He seems to be as near to total retreat from reality as he is capable.

With hindsight I must assume some responsibility for his need to retreat into that safe place. In the early days of learning about this illness I did not understand his increasing limitations, and with my lack of understanding I found myself pressing him to "do better." Even the mildest of pressure or impatience on my part were enough to catapult him over the edge, either into a flash of overt fury, or more commonly into his isolated place of refuge where there could be no expectations.

In my own defense I simply did not know yet. I think I was feeling that the closed eyes were shutting me out. Slowly

I began to understand. I am aware now, and in this ever changing scene I keep learning, little by little, to back off and to stop any attempt at verbal communication when the signs of stress appear. Usually, upon reassessing the situation, I find no need to get back to it. We wait awhile, and then we go on to other subjects when Dave is able.

I am aware that as time passes, communication on any level will no longer be an option. The decline will be inexorable. As I have learned other new disciplines I will learn this, also, but it will be one of the more difficult areas for me. Emotional vacuums, or attempts to cope with tentative circumstances within the family, are difficult areas for me. I enjoy interaction with people and find great rewards in just being a part of their lives. These are some of the things that are already changing, however.

Dave's growing isolation is becoming more obvious, and will be more and more a dominating factor for the two of us. As one becomes uncommunicative, the other becomes isolated, but hopefully our times of just communing will extend the bridge over that isolation gap, and give us a little more borrowed together-time.

But isolation need not necessarily mean aloneness for me, and when that feeling creeps in, almost overwhelmingly at times, I realize I must not give it permission. Regardless of what my emotions say to me, I know in my mind and heart that I am not alone now, nor will I be in the future. I am fortunate in having a wonderfully caring family, a warm and loving church, a host of caring friends, a most kind and competent doctor, and a God who knows we are here.

On occasion, a surge of ominous foreboding sweeps over me as I anticipate our as yet unexplored future. How will we make it? How will I handle the events that can, and most probably will, overtake us?

My response to these feelings is instinctive. I don't know how we will go about making it day by day, but thankfully it is not imperative that I know. Somehow, some way, we will make it in company with our God who does know, and who has been the third member of this team for nearly 60 years. And he isn't an absent, too-busy God, away out there in the great big bye-bye somewhere. He is right here in this reality of ours.

Psalm 46 starts off with the statement, "God is our refuge and strength, a very present help in trouble." This is His absolute promise. The Psalm says further, "Therefore we will not fear..." (KJV). Thus, my absolute objective is to trust and not be afraid. Even though there are times when I cannot see any light at the end of a long, long tunnel, there is no need that I should see: *I know He can!*

Unlike my friend's experience, Dave and I talk often and comfortably about Heaven, where hope and restoration abound, though that reality slowly becomes somewhat dimmed for Dave as his mental limitations take their toll.

As we continue to move on through this process known to me as the death of a mind, and as I inherit the results of the progressive aberrations of Alzheimer's, I am occasionally reminded of a comment by Dr. Paul Toms, former senior minister of Park Street Church in Boston. Dr. Toms reminded us that "while we are running around down here wringing our hands, God is not up there wringing His."

In confidence, though tested at times by human fragility, I keep on resting our case, moment by moment.

Chapter 9

COPING

Distress is defined in Webster's as "pain, anxiety and sorrow." Certainly then, Alzheimer's falls into the distress category, and as I reflect upon the subject I can apply each of these words to myself, and also to my husband, its victim. How could there not be distress -- pain, anxiety and sorrow, by an illness that changes, and eventually takes over, not only the life of a loved one but of that loved one's family as well.

I find myself challenged to somehow let that distress shape in me a positive reaction. The alternative would be to exist in quiet desperation. This, to my mind, would be a life not worth living at all. It would exhibit despair and resignation with grim determination, and with grimmer emotions. I, for one, cannot exist there. I am continually searching for the response God can help us make as we face a distressing situation, so that it doesn't completely alter whom we caregivers collectively, and I specifically, might wish to be.

God placed within me, for the most part, a love for people, a desire to laugh, to smile, to hug. I must find a way to protect the real me in the midst of stresses and frustrating changes. Melancholia and self-pity will not only drown my own spirit, but will make me into someone I won't like, and neither will anyone else!

In order to find my way it seems I must refine the art of coping. My love affair with the common dictionary led me to some provocative reflection on that little word. Consider its scope.

Coping implies a broad spectrum of propositions, call them ingredients, if you will. It can mean withstanding, tolerating, enduring; it can mean risking, suffering; it can involve grappling with, going up against, defying, making a stand, meeting head on, challenging, telling to one's face, confronting, holding at bay; it can also involve submitting or ignoring.

Last, but of greatest importance, are two more factors: abiding, and trusting. After any one or more of the diverse ingredients listed above may or may not have achieved their particular purposes, there is, for the Believer, the most important step in coping. That step is to abide and trust in Father and in His promise that *He will not give more than we can handle.*

These particular ingredients are probably the least popular in this day when any mention of God is, to many people, something a bit quaint and no longer relevant to our enlightened (?) state. After all, wasn't God declared dead a few decades ago by some portion of society? Those people do not even consider Him to be a factor; furthermore, to them, any dependence on Him, even if He was alive and well, would be considered a sign of weakness and inadequacy on their part.

But I would encourage any who do not buy the declaration concerning God's death, and who need to go beyond the ability to handle events in their lives all by themselves, not to succumb to that penchant for feeling weak and inadequate because you can't do it all by yourself. You were not meant to.

The tendency, however, is to withdraw into your little cocoon and enjoy your misery and desolation. I know. *I've been there.* It takes resoluteness to look up from the valleys, and with this illness valleys present themselves with increasing frequency. Handling them is an on-going process, and methods continually change.

Music often helps me when I recognize that tendency to feel desolate and alone. Just the words of one of the Gaither songs, "The God of the mountain is still God of the valley, the God of the day is still God in the night," have warmed my heart and turned it around so it could approach things with brightness and hope, again.

There are some of those valley days, however, that send me to my room to flop on my bed (and I use that word flop because that best describes just what I do!). I shed a few tears, and I cry, "Help!" Never has He failed to meet me there, not necessarily by changing the circumstances, but by giving me the assurance that He hears. Many times He has replaced my anguish with a refreshing calm.

He also assures me that it is O.K. to cry for myself. It is a part of the coping process, and He even reminds me that He has a special bottle in Heaven, just to keep my tears in (Ps. 56:8). Behold! With that realization a valley just became a peak! The great omnipotent God of creation cares that much for me. Selah! Think of that! I conclude that valley times become peak times when He is present.

As I attempt to make good decisions in handling the new and surprising incidents in our lives, I employ a variety of the above agenda for coping. More and more, however, I find myself learning to cope by ignoring. I try not to correct, find fault, act surprised or impatient, or show displeasure either verbally or with negative body language.

That is not an easy assignment for me. I find it difficult to stay in the right gear during abnormal circumstances. Any other approach, however, stimulates Dave's heavy sigh, followed by his dropping emotionally into that safe hole where there are no expectations, thus no failures. By using the ignoring factor we circumvent many of those awful feelings of isolation, inadequacy and depression which so easily sweep over him each time he realizes that his mind is not serving him as it once did.

Dave functions much of the time in a sea of blandness, both emotional and intellectual, and he does better when left there. He is no longer alert to either his capabilities, or his lack of them, and any attempts to reason through situations is futile. Someone very wisely said, "Don't try to reason with an Alzheimer's patient." I'm a slow learner. I tell myself that repeatedly, always with a bit of inner surprise. I don't seem quite ready to accept the extent to which reasoning is a lost quality between us.

I also need to constantly remind myself that any message, no matter how simple it may appear to me, is more and more a totally scrambled one to Dave. A request to bring the bag from the back seat of the car can end up by his bringing the umbrella from the trunk. Increasingly, all chores are becoming my responsibility.

The only constancy in the life of the Alzheimer's victim is the constancy of deterioration. Hope springs eternal, except here. All progress is downward into a void which becomes infinitely deeper and more inaccessible. And as the victim lives more and more in that lonely world, another lonely one is, at the same time, being carved out for the caregiver.

With this prospect, despair could reign except for the sure knowledge that the two of us, the victim who is lost in that awful void, and the mate who stands beside to care are not left to cope by ourselves. I must remember, always, that there are three of us here in this, our coping experience.

As I learn this art of coping, I know there will never come a time when I will have finally accomplished, once and for all, the goals of tranquility, composure, and appropriateness. There will be peaks and valleys, and mine will depend somewhat upon Dave's, all along the way. However, the peaks stand out, as peaks always do, and they present fleeting times of comfort to me. I doubt that Dave is aware of them.

I remember a trip through one of the mid-western plain states where I watched through binoculars for miles, wondering what that projection was on the distant horizon. It stood out conspicuously against the everlasting flatness of the surrounding terrain. As we finally drew close enough to determine its identity, it turned out to be a stand of trees around a farm house. It was only a small blip on that broad landscape, but it was a peak in the environment of the family who lived there, providing shade and protection from the elements, and a break in the sameness that surrounded them.

One morning Dave laughed out loud at an item on the TV news. I hadn't heard him laugh like that for a long time. It was a momentary blip, hardly a momentous event in a life. But that blip of laughter, though it probably would have gone unnoticed by others, was for me a peak, as it reached above the flat environment that can so dominate many Alzheimer's days. It was a bright and positive moment.

Gwen Bibber Kimball

Chapter 10

DETAILS

For some time now I have been concerned with my inability to settle down to quiet thoughtful extended prayer. My usual habit of prayer time each day, with a prayer list, seems to have become an almost impossible routine. After months of thought and fleeting guilt trips I have finally decided that the reason for my quandary lies within the realm of one rather simple word. That word is *Details*.

Details, details. My mind seems to be constantly challenged by details. They come from all directions and relate to all sorts of subjects. They run the gamut of managing a home; keeping a nurse's eye on a heart patient and dispensing medications; deciding which health management program we can afford and which best suits our needs (what could I or anyone else possibly know for sure about that subject?); handling normal and abnormal crises; taking care of bills, buying and preparing food; searching for lost hearing aids (I wish I could collect $1 an hour on that); and because of the need for those hearing aids I repeat everything in my life at least twice; turning off faucets which have been left running; watching to see that nothing, like lamps, get taken apart, etc., etc. Time and space prohibit an unabridged list.

And, oh yes, of course I must field that intrusion we call a telephone. Some nights I declare I am going to answer by saying, "Please excuse me for talking with my mouth full. My Mother did teach me it was not courteous, but you do know it is supper time?" Apparently telemarketers plan to call when they assume you will be there to answer. I am almost a convert of answering machines and caller I.D.'s.

The most compelling detail in my life is, "What is going on with my Dear One, where is he, and what is he doing now?" I need to be aware of his activities every minute he is awake, and at the same time intermingle that concern with all the other details that surround me.

For instance, the other afternoon I was using the sewing machine downstairs and I could hear his footsteps going around and around upstairs. I kept wondering what he was doing. Was he looking for something? What wouldn't I be able to find next time I looked, or what would I find when I finished my project and ventured to the floor above? My 77 year old knees don't clamor to do stairs unless they must, so I recklessly continued stitching, hoping the consequences would not be too distressing. Thankfully, all was well.

No matter where I am, or what I am doing, the story is always the same. If he is in the garage, what is he doing out there? Is something being put in the rubbish which should not be discarded? Or is something being put in a place where it is going to be damaged, or where I cannot possibly reach it, or even find it? Or is something being taken apart that will never go back together again? All of these have happened on more than one occasion.

We have a room we call, with much love and nostalgia, the Camp Room. We named it that because it reminds us of our old original family cottage in Maine where my brother and I spent the first five years of our lives. It has open rafters, (the better to hear the rain on the roof), and a beautiful old wood-burning stove which once provided the heat for that old cottage. Our Camp Room has 14 windows which look out into a completely private yard, lush in spring and early summer with rhododendrons and azaleas.

However, those 14 windows also have 14 screens which, of course, have to be stored in winter. They seem to manage to get stashed away routinely up overhead on the rafters of the garage where they become shelves for the next assortment of things that need to be stashed away because right now Dave is going through a neat stage. Everything has to be put somewhere, and if I am not watching, those screens can find their way to the rafters several times in one day.

To prevent having 14 sagging screens next spring I must check constantly, which means just about every time Dave is in the garage for any length of time. How he ever gets those screens up there is a mystery to me. You should see us trying to get them down. I am always wondering how I could handle such things in the spring if we don't take care of them now, because by then Dave may be beyond such activities.

My gardening tools get moved from their regular corner to anywhere he can put a nail or find an empty spot (which is usually a spot where I can't find them without a long search). At this juncture Dave considers all things *ours, or mine. There is no longer such a thing as yours.* As long as all things are ours he can put them wherever he wants, and use them however he wishes. My hand pruner became a wire cutter and now sports a big bite out of one blade. My new pruner is hidden.

I am sure his possessive attitude comes from the realization that he is losing control of family life and its decision-making processes. For that I have great understanding and compassion. But the pressure of the constant vigilance over details is not canceled out by mere understanding and compassion.

I found myself almost wishing for snow in October --
anything to cover up the last of the fallen leaves from our oaks
and maples. The lawn was being groomed day after day for
every stray leaf until we were beginning to have no grass.
Dave rakes with a heavy hand. I prevailed upon him to sweep
up the leaves with a light touch, which of course, he
remembered about 2 minutes.

Solution? The rakes are now hidden. Under my bed.
After several days of fruitless searching for them, which did
help occupy some of his time, he gave up and forgot about
raking. I said a quiet prayer of thanksgiving. Another detail
off my mind, at least for now.

I could go on, but you are probably asking, "Why are
you bothering to write all this down?" I'm writing this down
because we all need to realize that this is the way the days go,
these days of the caregiver. And we need to talk about it for
my sake, and for the sake of others who may be walking this
path thinking they are alone.

We also need to let well-meaning people know that we
are not dealing with just some ordinary memory loss "that we
all have as we get older." Don't say that, folks! I hear it all too
often. You haven't a clue, because my patient does not show
signs, publicly, of what is really going on at home. Trivial
comments are demeaning to a caregiver who is overloaded

with details too numerous to count, and who knows all too well that this is not just a case of getting older.

So, those details too numerous to count get me to the subject we started with. How does this all relate to prayer?

Let me tell you how it relates to my prayers. First, concerted prayer is hard work, and requires much emotional expenditure. It involves dealing again with details which by now are already reaching more than a bearable saturation point. The human mind, mine at least, has limitations, whereby I say, "Enough! Enough!" I cannot alter the demands of Dave's care, so I must amend other demands so as to arrive at a place where I can cope.

The Church, the religious community, traditions, etc., have all exerted tremendous pressures on the maintaining of one's prayer life, and I certainly would stress the importance of this vital ministry in the life of a Christian. But the why, and the how, for me, have become food for thought in these recent months.

As for the why, do we have other hidden purposes when we pray, aside from those worthy reasons which we know well? Are we attempting to please God? To placate our religious conscience? To gain brownie points? To feel spiritual -- sort of a "what a good girl am I" mentality?

And what about the how? Does this mean eyes shut, hands folded, prayer list out, people and their needs addressed in detail by an already overcrowded mind? What about the situations in life that have already caused time and energy to run out, even before all of this is added? And please don't quote priorities to caregivers. Their priorities are established, with little or no chance for change or rearrangement.

What does God mean when He says to pray without ceasing? Some days every breath seems to be a prayer: of thanksgiving; for patience; for direction; for wisdom; for someone's need. Is this the real meaning of praying without ceasing for me at this time in my life, with routine prayer time not eliminated, merely curtailed, and verbiage abbreviated?

As I grappled with these questions there slowly dawned upon me a new awakening. It was rich, comforting, and totally fulfilling. I am realizing that my once regular, scheduled Bible and prayer time is being rearranged by circumstances beyond my control, at the insistence of that robber of everything that is normal: Alzheimer's. I am sensing more and more God's Holy Spirit graciously attending me, where I am, all the time, taking my concerns, even my thoughts, and presenting them to my Father for me. After all, how many details does He need me to tell Him if He even knows when the sparrow falls?

With this realization comes the true understanding of praying without ceasing for this time in my life. How satisfying, settling, and supportive that is to me. The awareness of His continuous intercession in my life, as He promised, has set me free -- free not only to walk away from my legalistic guilt, but free to find adequacy in my necessarily restructured prayer time.

Chapter 11

A TRUST

The care of my husband through the course of that illness known as Alzheimer's took on a totally new meaning one day when I concluded, after much pondering, that the God who doesn't do mean things to people, but does allow human infirmities, has entrusted to me this crisis experience. I deduce that something that has been entrusted to someone indeed becomes a trust.

To consider Alzheimer's a trust stands in stark contrast to the opinion held by some that unpleasant events in ones life are necessarily matters of judgment and punishment. Neither Dave nor I have ever placed this affliction in such a category. We are content with His purpose. Our desire is that its impact upon our lives might in some way bring encouragement to others who find themselves with the same struggles. Thus, one of the reasons for writing this book.

Needless to say, trust was hardly the term I had previously had in mind as I assessed this intruder, and I must admit that I occasionally lose sight of that designation. When that happens and I find I am out of control, I ask myself with some disdain, "What happened to that trust?" I get back on track by reminding myself of my conviction when I was feeling more sane, sensible and reasonable.

Even on the most difficult days I find I cannot disengage myself from that conviction, although it may take several reminders. It is a galvanizing element in my daily walk, and it wraps itself around me like a supportive cloak. It has to be something that God placed in my heart. It has nothing to do with my being noble.

I do keep the subject of burn-out in mind. Our professional people never let me lose sight of that factor. I am confident I will know when it is time to turn this trust over to professional caregivers. That time usually does come for most of us, although my desire would be that Dave could go to sleep, for the last time, in his own bed. I assume we all desire that, even for ourselves.

Our friend Larry, an Alzheimer's sufferer and a major personality in my book, "You Say WHAT, Lord?", died at home. His wife Barbara, who had cared for him the entire way, said it was such a comfort to slip into his empty but still warm bed the night he died, to start her grieving process as she slept where he had so recently lain. What an uncommon Lady!

This trust of ours will increasingly be mine to manage by myself, with the aid of family. That makes it a new discipline in the lives of two people who have previously functioned as a team. We will always be a team, Dave Kimball and I, but the roles are now changed, and the responsibilities are reversed.

As for family, they are irreplaceable in the process. In my opinion there needs to be a huge reawakening to the sense of responsibility of the young generation toward the family unit. We are such a fractured society. Grandparents and their needs must be rebuilt into our family communities. All too many Grammies and Grampies are like out-of-date commodities, no longer useful, stashed away in holding areas and forgotten. This was one situation my husband hoped to address when he founded the Community Chaplain Service.

To return to our trust and its impact upon my life, I find myself viewing it from several directions, three in particular.

The first one is the humility I feel as I contemplate what apparently must be God's confidence in me as He permits this challenge to be mainly mine. I know that any success on my part will be realized only as I learn to depend upon a strength beyond myself. He surely never expected me to handle this all alone. My heart goes out to any caregivers who are not in touch with a God whom they are positive knows them and loves them.

Years ago I learned a poem to present in a public speaking class. It has always been a favorite of mine and I have never forgotten it. Appropriately it says:

> *"Child of my love, lean hard*
> *And let me feel the pressure of your care;*
> *I know your burden, child, I shaped it;*
> *Poised it in My own hand,*
> *Made no proportion in its weight to your unaided*
> *strength;*
> *For even as I laid it on I said,*
> *'I shall be near, and while she leans on me,*
> *This burden shall be Mine, not hers.'*
> *So shall I keep my child in the encircling arms*
> *of My own love.*
> *Here lay it down, nor hesitate to impose it on a*
> *shoulder which upholds the government of worlds.*
> *Yet closer come; you are not near enough;*
> *I would embrace your care so that I might feel My child*
> *reposing on my breast.*
> *You love Me? I knew it. Doubt not, then;*
> *But loving Me, lean hard."*
> Author Unknown

I do find that at times it would be much easier for me to run, than to lean. Nevertheless, how good of God to understand, and in consideration of my humanness to invite me to Himself as in Matthew 11:28,29. He says there, "Come unto me all ye that labor and are heavy laden and I will give you rest. Take my yoke upon you and learn of me ... and ye shall find rest unto your souls." (KJV) Herein I attempt to rest, hindered not by any inadequacy of His, only of mine.

The second thought of mine was one of fear, fear of my lack of patience. I know myself, and this gives me trouble. The challenge to any caregiver's patience, 36-hour day* after 36-hour day, week after week, is formidable. For one like me who has struggled all her life to be a patient person, it is scary. I move and think quickly and have had to learn not to expect others to do the same. Now, here I am, facing this unbelievable challenge, mainly a test of patience, as Dave's thought processes, movements, reasoning, understanding, even hearing, become progressively slowed, and his emotions become undependable.

I shared my sense of need for patience one day years ago with our beloved family physician, Dr. Frank Rubin who had attended the birth of our daughters and had seen us through several surgical experiences. He reminded me that half of the battle was already won just by my being aware of the need.

Imagine that! Half the battle won! Already! In my youth and inexperience I felt elated that so much progress had been made that easily.

I did not share those unrealistic impressions with Dr. Rubin. I am sure he would have smiled gently at my naivete. But I have thought of that comment of his many times. It stands out like a landmark. In spite of my unrealistic evaluation of it at the time, it did help me to realize that if I had not recognized the need there would have been no starting point.

I must confess to having been quite impressed with myself for my noble insight into my need. Such candid self-evaluation would warrant God's answering my prayer speedily, I was quite sure. I've learned since, during the nearly six decades of my Christian life, that God has His own method and time schedule in answering our prayers.

Back there, as a twenty-year-old, I expected immediate action, because I knew all the good verses about "ask and you shall receive", etc. He would somehow produce a tray complete with the fruit of the Spirit, and from it I could just take and eat. It would just be all that simple, and that would be the end of the subject.

I soon learned it was not all that simple, and it was not the end of the subject. I had not spent much time on the "wait patiently" verses, waiting not being one of the favorite pastimes of the young and the restless. I did find, however, that my much needed fruit of the Spirit was, and is, there for the taking, but there was no tray. Instead, I simply became more and more aware of my need. Disarming.

As my elation rapidly deteriorated, I found I was just beginning the struggle that would ensue for the remainder of my life. Any accomplishment I attained as I attempted to achieve this goal of patience came, not by God's handing it to me, but by my taking of it through practice, practice, practice, like an athlete preparing for the Olympics. In and out of the pool, on and off the track, over and over on the ice. This Alzheimer's thing mandates my ultimate in practice time for acquiring patience, and will be without question my Olympic experience.

Whether or not I will ever stand on the podium and receive a medal for patience under duress is a moot question. If so, I fear it will not be the Gold.

My third thought had to do with the guilt trip I could be on if I did not attain my goals. That, I believe, will be up to me entirely -- whether or not I will permit myself to fall into that trap. If I do so, it will be in part because I will expect perfection of myself and will permit myself no failures. I refuse to do that, even though in some areas I do tend to be a perfectionist.

The Apostle Paul, in Romans 7:15, addressed the struggle within himself and referred to "not doing those things which he wanted to do." However, he did not continue to bewail that wretched state but claimed grace in Jesus Christ. That grace is mine, also, and will always be there for me, all the while allowing me my humanness with its room to fail.

After all, pole-vaulters don't make every high jump, skaters fall, little gymnasts do poorly and dissolve into tears, divers hit their heads, and skiers know the agony of defeat. All is not victory all the time. But they pick themselves up, dust themselves off, and head out to try again. As for the number of times I have done just that, we won't even go there!

Mercifully, Dave forgets my lapses of grace in a minute or two, at times even before I can say, "I'm sorry." If there are any blessings in memory loss this has to be one of them. How providential for this caregiver.

So go my days, satisfied with my progress most of the time as I attempt to handle this trust, allowing myself some failures, and most of all, ever learning, on this new road that Dave and I have not traveled together until now.

* From the title of the book, "The 36 Hour Day", by Nancy L. Mace, M.A., and Peter V. Rabins, M.A., M.P.H.

Gwen Bibber Kimball

Chapter 12

HUMOR

I have been feeling onslaughts on my reservoir of patience for some time now. Dave's definite diagnosis of Alzheimer's has caused me to examine that reservoir and to begin to look for outlets that would help me to let off pressure.

Endurance seems to be the most fragile at the end of a long day, and the erosion of that endurance can easily eventuate in an emotional collision between the caregiver and the patient. Because there is already little capacity for reasoning, collisions are destined to be nonproductive. Not only are they nonproductive, they become counter productive, and they represent an enormous demand on one's self-control.

This is an ever-learning situation in a totally new area, for two people one of whom is no longer capable of further learning. In spite of my awareness of the need to develop patience all along the way, pressurized situations do appear, and I must find ways to keep them from becoming overheated. That seems, at times, to be a gigantic problem. I have looked for answers over and over, and have searched for every possible way to handle issues with restraint. Among other outlets, I have discovered one we are apt to overlook for whatever reason, perhaps in the name of human dignity. That is the outlet of humor.

What is humor? Webster says it is "an expression of mirth or merriment, and can be the result of the bringing together of incongruities which arise naturally due to some certain situation." Webster must have known all about Alzheimer's, because if ever there were incongruities arising out of certain situations, the life of an Alzheimer's patient is going to present those certain situations!

Somewhere in the process of this illness I had to make a decision. Are we to consider every incident as so sad, and so tragic, that we must do nothing but grieve? Or can we be a bit easy on ourselves, and look for some humor, at least in the earlier stages before this illness makes its full impact? Even at that time I suspect humor will have a place. Dave and I are not there yet, so that remains to be seen.

For now, one of my safety valves will be the employing of some merriment on a day that is bleak, and believe me, those bleak days do come. I am convincing myself that many experiences are neither so private, nor so sacrosanct, that we can't brighten their bleakness with a chuckle.

This may take some retraining of my natural reactions, but in the name of survival I must try. After all, our brief visit here upon this earth is only a visit. There is no reason for us to treat it as if there were no glorious future out ahead that will set us free from these events which so violate who we are down here.

I am trying to replace feelings of frustration with casual, kind, loving humor. I could have handled many situations so much more graciously had I learned a bit earlier that this is the best my loved one can do, give a hug or a pat with a chuckle, and get on with life.

If I sense that Dave cannot make light of a situation and I need to laugh, I can always share it with my trusted friend, Joan, who will laugh with me but do so with love and respect for Dave.

One day when Dave was showing frustration we suggested to him that there were two people living in his skin. One was named Dave, and the other was named Al, short for Alzheimer's. When Dave does something that is decidedly unconventional, or that expresses a thought that doesn't quite make it, we remind him that "that's Al again; don't pay too much attention to him." That very often ends the subject without getting into a corrective mode, which only creates confusion for Dave and goes nowhere except into frustration for everyone.

Trying to change Al's mind is literally like bouncing a ball off a cement wall. The subject never changes, it just keeps coming back at you. You learn to let it go after the first bounce and hope that Al will not pursue it further.

Sometimes Al is persistent. An example: Dave often does not get his car door shut completely. The red light on the dash says "door open."

"Honey, try reclosing your door. It isn't quite shut."

"What?"

"Try reclosing your door. It isn't quite shut."

"My door is shut," says Dave with finality. I recognize Al.

"I don't believe it can be, because my red light is on."

"What?"

Repeat.

Ignoring the proof, Al insists his door is shut. "It must be your door," he replies.

At this point I cajole. I open and close my door. "The light is still on. Just try opening and closing yours and see if the light goes out."

Al responds with a heavy sigh, grudgingly opens his door with an obviously annoyed thrust, and then shuts it more firmly than necessary.

I respond with, "Oh good, the light just went off."

Al sulks in silence for a few miles. Shortly, Dave returns and doesn't even remember the incident.

This will recur often. Unfortunately my only other choice would be to turn off the motor, take the keys with me, force my 79-year-old-knees out of the car in spite of their objections, walk around the car and close his door myself. The first option seems to be the easier solution, although I would prefer not to stimulate Al's pouting and sulking. But that's Al, and as I said, we try not to pay too much attention to him. We just wait until he goes away, and not let his little incidents ruffle the surface and spoil a whole day, especially if it is one of those sore spot things that could so easily become a major focus.

Is it habit, ethnic background or rearing? What is it that makes some folks forever fragile and melancholy? Every event in their lives seems to be doleful. Again I am reminded of my desire for God to give me a merry heart and a cheerful countenance, both for myself and for those who are around me. The people in my life who have been inspirations have never been the ones with the sad eyes and the turned down mouths.

I had an elderly friend years ago whom I lovingly called "Blue Jay". He sat endlessly rocking in his chair, moaning to himself over and over, "Oh dear, dear, dear, dear, dear," (always five times), always finalized with a huge sigh, and always repeated momentarily, on and on... Deliver me! Strangely, this man had a tremendous sense of humor. He could be wonderfully funny, but he had let some sad events in his life produce that morbid attitude, and most of the time it took charge of who he was.

I have learned that the events which seem so desolate today can be the things about which you'll say in a few years, "You won't believe this one, and it really happened!" We experienced this on numerous occasions in our thirty years in the pastorate because, you know, even Christians forget the Golden Rule. Sometimes there is only one thing to do with your agony and that is to mix it with the knowledge that one day you can, and will, laugh about it, even if only at its absurdity.

I have told many young pastors' wives never to lose their sense of humor. This also goes for the Alzheimer's caregiver, and here I am again, after all these years, rehearsing that same message. Now, however, it is a re-run to myself.

Let me give you an example: Karen and I returned from shopping one day, perhaps two years or more ago, the day I found I could no longer leave Dave alone, even for short periods.

I noticed that my flower pots needed watering so I took my watering can to the hose for a refill. No water! I checked the source. Faucet on. I then went to my rather complicated hub which connected hoses going to different locations around the yard. They were not only disconnected, they had been cut apart, obviously with a sharp knife, (Dave's pocket knife?), and all those connectors were just lying there, scattered around on the ground. They seemed to be telling me that there was indeed more than one way to disconnect a hose.

I couldn't believe what I was seeing. My first reaction was to be more than mildly incensed *because I was still not willing nor able to admit to myself that my husband was incapable of thinking any better than this.*

Furthermore, to connect those hoses so they didn't leak had been a challenge for this seventy-five year old, and I was not anxious to have to do it all over again.

I began to feel symptoms of savoring a decisive confrontation. Karen, being a very perceptive young lady, read my mind. Before I became too articulate she came to me, put her arms around me and said, "Lady", (a pet name since her childhood), "it's not going to get better, you know. It's going to get worse."

Then she asked me, "Mom, do you remember the story Tony told you of the man with Alzheimer's who couldn't remember how to raise the venetian blinds in his bedroom? He went to the basement, found the tin snips, returned to his room, cut said blinds straight up the middle and proceeded to tie them back like draperies, with pieces of string. Do you remember that, Mom?"

I remembered. My fury turned to something bordering on hysteria. We laughed together 'til my tears came, and with a big hug and a pat on the back she sent me off to do the repair job on my hoses.

Humor saved my day, and I have thought back over that incident many times since, each time experiencing those same liberating feelings. It is now a sort of traffic signal to me. When things have a tendency to get out of hand and my lights turn red, the venetian blinds become a hook I try to remember to hang my attitude on.

Chapter 13

TEARS

Sometimes I cry. Not often. Just sometimes. Tears have not consumed large portions of my life. We Mainers are perceived as somewhat stiff-upper-lip folks, a perception which is apt to depict us as being cold and unemotional. As in all locales, we have our percentage of those whose upper-lip does always seem to be stiff, but most of us are not so much unemotional as we are discriminatory about the why, and the how long, of our indulgence.

Perhaps environment plays a part. Let me digress here for a bit and explain to you what it was like to grow up as a down-east Maine Yankee in a very remote area.

Maine as I knew it in the twenties and thirties did not lend itself to an undisciplined, cry-baby attitude about life. By comparison with today's standards it was a spartan existence, offering few of the luxuries we now take so for granted and think we can't possibly live without.

I never fail to be totally mystified by the morning shower that rules lives. Daughter Karen recounted the story of a co-worker who called in to say she could not come to work because her electricity had gone off during the night and she had no hot water for her shower. Now, HONESTLY! Indeed, trials are relative. I keep that in mind, even as Dave and I walk daily through a considerable one called Alzheimer's. It will be worse.

Speaking of that near-sacred morning shower, I remember commenting once in the presence of our girls that I never took a bath in a bathtub until I was 17, when I went away to school...to which they replied, aghast, "MOTHER!" Cleanliness was arrived at via a basin of water each day, and the galvanized washtub each Saturday night, with only enough water of varying temperatures to accomplish the job at hand. A deterrent to a deep soak in a nearly full tub was the reminder that all that water had to be carried by someone, pail by pail, from the Lake, as was our experience when we lived at Camp with our mother and grandparents when we were very small. Camp was a summer cottage which was our year-round home from the time of our birth, a place of very deep roots for both my brother Harry (better known as Bud) and me.

When we moved into town for schooling, water came from a neighbor's well, or from the town pump if there was no water on the place -- and we had no water on the place. At a fairly early age, 8 and 9 or so, we were carrying enough buckets on wash day to fill two wash tubs and the copper boiler atop the kitchen range. Daily the drinking water bucket had to be kept filled. Neither one of us was especially enthusiastic about the whole idea, but I don't remember that it ever occurred to us to complain about it, nor did it seem unusual in any way. That's the way things were for nearly everyone who lived there.

Although those early days at Lake Pennamaquan were sparce -- no electricity, no furnace, no running water, no indoor bathroom, no telephone, and of course no car, we remember them as wonderful. We felt no need for anything we didn't have.

Providing transportation for us children were two legs with feet bare in summer, shoes of varying degrees of protection the rest of the year, and snow shoes added when the going got really rough. Grandpa had us on snowshoes when we were three years old, so says his diary. The adults, of course, did without the bare feet. All else was the same. The nearest Post Office was two miles down the Maine Central Railroad, Bangor to Calais line. Did you ever walk the tracks? They give no choices. They are either slippery in winter or torrid in summer, and at best they provide an awkward-gaited unrhythmical trek.

Dr. Best was 5 miles away by horse. Only major health crises warranted getting to him. Family members never seemed to panic at handling some of the simple things that today end up in the Emergency Room. Neither of us children saw Dr. Best until we were five and six years of age.

Just picture those early days in that one-room cottage at the Lake, three adults, two babies fifteen months apart in ages (sans Pampers). Grampa carried water from the Lake for all utility purposes such as washing all those diapers, doing dishes, taking baths, etc., in winter necessitating a hole cut in the ice, of course. Also, the spring, a pool of clear pure water nestled under a clump of trees on the hillside, had to be chopped open each morning, and enough water carried to accommodate cooking and drinking for the day.

Work at the woodpile in all temperatures was a constant for Grampa almost all year, and on the coldest nights in winter he had to crawl out of his cozy bed to keep that stove going. Imagine waking up in a -30 something degree temperature and the fire out!

Winter saw Nana knitting and crocheting in her spare time, whatever of that commodity she had, and she and

Grampa calling on neighbors, none of them nearby. Often the temperature was below zero, and Nana's height at 5 feet 1/2 inch only slightly topped the depth of the snow at times. Snowshoes for both were a must.

In the Summer there was the wonderful garden from which we ate sumptuously. Blueberries and raspberries grew all around us and had to be picked. When I was old enough I had to help. How I hated that, but the rule was that those who didn't pick berries didn't eat berries.

My brother exhibited more berry-picking talent than I and was down at the Lake sailing his boats, his quota filled, while I wandered all over the berry patch looking for the big ones. Eventually I learned!

Hordes of minges, black flies, and mosquitoes always descended upon us just as the weather improved. When I am there now, as an indulged adult, I can't imagine how we ever coped with them. But gardens got planted, and the regular chores necessary to life there were carried out, regardless.

There were no sophisticated aero-spray cans for protection from those hungry predators. What was available Nana called "skeeter-scoot," and it was dispensed from a hand-manipulated sprayer with a push handle and it was used sparingly. Money was not spent on anything that could be considered a luxury. A simpler, cost free solution when one of those pests came whining around, usually just before daybreak, was not to get up and light a kerosene lamp and institute a search, but to bare a small area of skin, and leave a hand ready for action. When you could feel the air from its wings you pounced on the intruder with a resounding slap and went back to sleep, feeling smugly satisfied. During the day you just coped, and when they were at their worst, at dusk, all activity took place indoors behind screens.

Nothing was wasted there. Produce not eaten was canned in preparation for the long winter. We were never asked what we would eat. We just ate. Bread was homemade, wonderful with fresh strawberries with a little sugar, crushed over a hot heel. But after the second day and that bread became a bit dry, as all homemade bread does, I silently vowed to myself I would never eat bread when I grew up, even if it was "the staff of life and everything else was only there to help it go down more easily," which was Nana's dismal opinion. When we moved into town and on occasion ran out of bread I thought I was in Heaven when I could go to the store and buy a loaf of store bread!

However, having to pick my share of berries, and dealing with homemade bread not withstanding, I hardly remember an unhappy day there at the Lake. Hardy as life was, there was a lot of love and caring, and we both remember feelings of security. I presume those feelings were fostered in large part by the real parenting we received from the adults in our lives, in spite of an absent father. Grampa in a total sense was my dad.

Nana and Grampa were stout-hearted people who had weathered their own crises. They had lost their baby son at age six. I'm sure they cried over that. Their pain over Mother's divorce must have been deep because they placed supreme value upon the family unit.

Nana occasionally took a walk down a wooded path and I recall her weeping softly as she disappeared from sight into quiet privacy. I was not as distressed by the fact of her tears as I was concerned over the reason for them, because I was sure Nana only cried over important things. When she emerged from her quiet place she cheerfully got on with life, and this little child learned that there are some things in life about which even adults must cry.

Grampa's diaries reveal no feelings of self-pity or of deprivation, he who had come, from choice, from a lovely home in Eastport complete with all the comforts of furnace heat, running water, etc. There is no mention of misery, nor do I read of, or remember any complaining. Life, complete with its challenges, was basically good, God was good. In each life there had to be some pain and discomfort. That was not a choice. But allowing it to generate constant annoyance and distress was a choice, and that choice was not to be indulged in.

My Mother was an incredibly talented woman, an early divorcee in days when being a divorced woman was neither acceptable nor fashionable. She found herself faced with the challenge of earning a living for herself and her two children, not a casual responsibility in that day. She must have had her times of tears, dauntless though she was, but as a child I never saw them.

Yet, when I on occasion seemed to feel the need to cry, her advice to me was, "If you need to cry, have your cry, and then get on with life." That seemed to sum up the Maine philosophy for handling adversity. I remember feeling comforted that it was O.K. for me to cry, but I also remember taking seriously her suggestion that there was a time to cry, a time to stop crying, and a time to move on.

Our adults left us with a legacy of adaptability, resilience, and courage, the memories of which still influence me to this day, especially as Dave and I attempt to handle the crises emanating from the presence of Alzheimer's in our lives.

One day on a dark December morning Dave was up at 5:45. He dressed and went directly out to the yard -- to pick up his twigs. It was only just becoming light so he had to bend low to see them. Picture the scene, and my feelings, as I looked out the window at this College Valedictorian man of mine. Softly I said, "How sad," and I cried briefly, the first time in a long while I've shed tears over the twig subject.

My frustration over his progressive deafness is intensified by the increased repetition I must employ in order for us to communicate even over the simplest of subjects. Sometimes I weep in sheer weariness of voice and spirit.

In Dave's world, what happened five minutes ago is gone from his mind, and it is increasingly impossible for me to explain anything clearly or simply enough for a message to register. The receptors have simply ceased working.

His frustration over his lack of memory and his inability to reason cause him to explode into episodes of anger, name calling and door slamming. These outbursts still shock me initially, and long-term they become a catalyst to my emotions. The futility of the situation presents the need for an outlet for me, and that outlet on occasion is tears of utter desolation while I regain my emotional balance and move on, to focus on Alzheimer's rather than on the responses of its victim.

Along the way I was encouraged by well-meaning and caring friends to try vitamins and/or herbal supplements which were billed to help slow the process of Alzheimer's. Nothing promised any significant amount of actual improvement.

I pondered the subject very seriously. This was a heavy-hearted time for me, but I finally came to the conclusion that it would show neither love nor kindness to do anything that would prolong Dave's existence in his present state. If it couldn't help decisively, was it fair to add any time to his struggle? That option seemed to me to be no option at all.

I decided to let things run their course and be over sooner than later, for Dave's sake. With Heaven as a bright promise straight from Father, then the sooner the better. My confidence in Heaven left me no need for tears here. Only a sad heart.

But, as I said, sometimes I do cry -- from sadness, frustration, aggravation or even fury. I don't cry long. Usually it is just a brief "I do feel so sorry for myself" interlude, but each time I sense a release in my spirit when those flood gates open.

Aside from my early training for the need for some brevity to my weeping, I have an added incentive: the longer I cry the redder my eyes and nose get, especially my nose, and there is always that lurking fear that sure enough, someone is going to ring that doorbell and find me looking *like this!* It would seem that sometimes just a touch of vanity helps save a day.

Gwen Bibber Kimball

Chapter 14

MY ORGAN RECITAL

Now, prepared to be bored. Who wants to listen to someone's "organ recital" about their ill-health? Probably a large percentage of you know of those people whom you glimpse from a distance and deliberately avoid meeting, because it will be good for half an hour of operations, doctors and medications. I am now joining those ranks. My attention to Dave's impairment was recently interrupted by a wholly unexpected descent onto a new plateau of my own. Thus this recital.

I had never entertained the slightest thought that I might, in some way, become physically incapable of caring for Dave on a daily basis. I have been a very active person with no disabilities except the general problems of aging joints, and a slight slowing down of my usual pace. A shot of Cortisone for an occasionally painful hip plus the care of a good Orthopedist seemed to keep me going at the pace necessary. (I told you this would be boring.) I have tried to monitor my activities to correspond to this slight impairment, though I have gained the reputation, by some family members, of being one of those 'don't stop 'til you drop' Yankees. However wisely or unwisely I have accomplished it, I have always enjoyed handling the demands of both home and yard.

Recently my wisdom was overcome by that certain enthusiasm which emerges in the springtime when gardens are beginning to exhibit their first signs of life beyond winter. Yard lovers anticipate this awakening all during the snow and the cold. But there are always those left-over leaves from last year that seem determined to hang onto the trees defiantly 'til deep winter storms and winds bring them down. Their presence inhibits every attempt the plants make to emerge and do what they are supposed to do. We wonder, each spring, why they couldn't have fallen and been raked up along with all the others. Instead, here they are! Even the grass is stifled in its efforts to assert itself because of the layers and mounds of leaves that lie all over the place.

Obviously, rake we must, again. And of course, instead of busying myself cautiously for half an hour or so, my or so became three and a half hours. After all, it was good healthy exercise out in the warm sun and fresh air. No lifting, no straining. I forgot the twisting. I forgot the dormant state of muscles after a long winter. I also forgot my age.

When I was a child my grandfather called me a "strammer," his word for people who were ever on the move, and who usually had their feet off the ground. He despaired that I would ever be a lady. His most often-repeated request of me was, "Heavens, Gwen, put your feet down!" We joked in later years that "heavens" was Grampa's strongest swear word.

I once stated to my mother that some of my friends sure were popular with the boys and her response was, "If you'd take off those blue jeans and get off that bicycle the boys might know you're a girl!"

My Maine-born Uncle Lewis once stated in his typical manner, "Judas priest, she runs like a deer," and I must confess to doing everything possible to keep up with my big brother who was only fifteen months older than I. Through the years, however, society in general and my role as a pastor's wife in particular modified my propensity for much of that tomboy activity. I have wished that Grampa could know that eventually I did become able, when necessary, to be a lady, and without too much pain; however, our girls have said many times, "Slow down, Mother, we can feel the breeze!"

But back to the leaves. After they were bagged it was still warm and beautiful outside, so true to form, I moved on. I went into my beloved Shady Garden and there I gave the ladies' slippers, bleeding hearts, trilliums, etc., breathing space as I cleaned up more winter debris. I just had to do it, of course, because -- why -- the trilliums had buds ready to open! They just couldn't be left as they were, and besides, I really didn't feel tired. So much for the compelling presence of energy, enthusiasm, and lack of good judgment!

Next morning my enthusiasm was less vibrant when I found I could not bear weight on my left hip. My confidence, as I pondered my state, rested in my conviction that in a couple of days all would be well, so I hobbled around holding onto furniture, did what I had to, and waited.

But I was not functioning better in two days. Discomfort was increasing, sleep was sketchy, and any movement made me grimace in pain. Fear began to descend. All sorts of questions blazed in front of me. What if I had to deal with this, long-term? What of the work involved in caring for the house, the yard, and most of all in caring for Dave and knowing where he was every minute? How to grocery-shop in our huge super-markets where the milk is as far away from the entrance as one can possibly get; how to go down the stairs to do the laundry, which always involves coming back up again, of course. For some years now I have told Dave, "If you want to keep me in the cellar forever just take the railing off the stairs," always said as a big joke, or course. Now it was more reality than joke, because I could not get up those stairs even with the railing.

I slowly let myself settle into a state of panic. This was a totally new experience for me. I do not panic easily. But even my prayers were panic-filled. "Lord, how could you let this happen to me," became my peevish and petulant prayer over and over again. I completely ignored the thought that my own poor judgment might possibly be a factor.

I was so bewildered, and I felt so alone. It seemed that I was the only one in the entire universe who was aware that I had a problem of this magnitude. Not true, of course, but the feelings were starkly real. Those feelings were partly my own fault. I had not told the girls. Michelle was recovering from a broken elbow, and Karen was two hours away by car. And, I rationalized, both of them were busy with their own lives.

Normally Dave would have been my right-hand man, but that is now all in the past. I must make adjustments to his almost total unawareness of reality. Every day it was the same dialogue. "Is there something wrong?", he would ask, upon seeing me creep around at an entirely different pace from my usual one. "I have a problem with my hip, Dear." "Have you seen the Doctor?" "Yes." He had, of course, accompanied me there. "How did this happen?" "Is it something new?" "Is there something you can do for it?", over and over again, which in itself took its toll on patience and composure. I not only had no answer for him, I could not reveal to him my feelings of devastation as they related to him. He could not possibly handle them. My sense of aloneness was suffocating.

For many months I had ended my evening with one of my many Gaither videos, singing and clapping along softly, a happy and confident way to put my day to rest. Now I wanted no part of singing and clapping. I simply could not warm up to "When Jesus says It's Enough It Will Be Enough." Enough was right now, please!

I seemed to have moved into a bleak realm that prohibited me from feeling any hope. Anything that interrupts the ability to give the constant care and attention required by a mate with Alzheimer's can produce panic, and I panicked. I wasn't accustomed to those feelings. For two days and nights I remained unable to move, emotionally, from that morass. Satan had a field-day with my vulnerable areas, and I cooperated with him by forgetting temporarily Who, indeed, was in charge. It was a dark night experience.

My most troubling area was the responsibility for Dave's future. I realized more fully than ever before that the quality of Dave's life depended on me. Would he have to be deposited into a nursing home somewhere because I was not going to be able to do what was necessary to care for him at home? How could I ever tell him that...

A variety of subjects began to press in upon me. To go straight to Heaven would be so easy and wonderful, but should escape be the major purpose for desiring to go there? Was the alternative to be the transplanting of one, or maybe both of us, into a long-term care facility to waste away in a geri-chair for who knows how long? That was unthinkable. It was one of my darkest times, but it did afford me a long look into the world of those who have had to do just that. I must admit to a much greater empathy for them than I had ever experienced before.

My literal feeling in the middle of those lost days was one of frantically waving my hand and calling, "Yoo-hoo, Lord, I am down here. Did You forget about me?"

How could I have pondered that thought for a single moment! Hadn't He placed a sufficient curiosity in the heart of this little five-year-old girl to cause her to keep asking people who Jesus really was, and why He died (even though no one seemed to know)?; and hadn't He kept that mild, though persistent, curiosity alive 'til that little girl was seventeen years old?; and hadn't He seen to it that at that time she *happened* to move to a place where a faithful Pastor preached a message which answered her question and she could respond joyously,

"Why, of course! He is God and He died in my place!?" How much more proof did I need that He had not, and would not, "forget me!" Back there I was just one more little five-year-old in this great big world; yet I had His individual attention. Why would I not have it now?

Forgetting Who is in charge of our lives and Who has the answers had reduced me to wringing my hands! I thought I knew better than that.

Chapter 15

WHOSE WE ARE

When I remembered to let God remind me Whose I am, and Who is in charge, I learned something that does not come easily for some of us old Yankees. I had to relinquish my independence and become willing to rely upon family and friends for hands-on support. I learned also that actually becoming helpless is quite different from merely contemplating helplessness. But first and foremost I realized that I must return to my reliance upon my God. It seems I keep learning things I thought I already knew.

Of course, the same good God who has followed my life so closely all these years had already seen my need and was planning on my behalf. His first step in meeting that need and getting me out of my slough of despond was seeing to it that I received a phone call from Karen. She heard the distress in my voice immediately and said, "What's going on, Mom?" I tried to tell her my dilemma. As soon as she heard she said, "I have sick time for family crises. I'll be right there." She was here in two hours. Michelle would have been here already, had I let her know. Karen wasted no time calling her.

When Karen walked in the back door that day my world opened up again. I hadn't realized how much I needed someone to take charge for me. That realization freed my emotions which had been locked up so tightly. I was finally able to cry. It was safe now, because here was someone who could handle my tears. Dave could not.

Hope began to return. It seemed as if the sun came out. My natural optimism made its appearance. I thanked God repeatedly that His care was visible once again. I realized that I was the one who had limited Him by not letting my family know I needed them. Neither Michelle nor Karen was too happy with me.

Now we would get on with that wonderful managed care of which I had reluctantly, though hopefully, become a part. Wrong. A visit to the Orthopedist was approved, but without an x-ray. In my limited opinion I deemed an x-ray to be as important to an Orthopedist as a cardiogram was to a Cardiologist. Apparently that also was wrong.

After nearly two weeks, on a Friday, I was finally given permission for an x-ray, but found I would have to wait 'til after the weekend to get permission to have it read by someone other than my own Orthopedist who was by now on vacation.

Karen decided the system was not working too well and insisted she take me to the Emergency Room for medical help which included x-rays, and something for pain so I could sleep at night. I was glad to pay out-of-pocket for the privilege of some care.

The diagnosis? No problem, the pain notwithstanding.

Michelle helped me with renting crutches, an item you can believe I embraced with vigorous mental and vocal objections, and with much embarrassment. ME on crutches? Unthinkable!

A month after my injury, during which time I freed myself from my HMO dictatorship, and was able to see my Orthopedist with x-rays in hand, he initially thought of a stress crack in the femur, but it was finally determined that I was suffering from a severe tendonitis. Eventually, with pain medication, the crutches, ice packs, and rest from activity, I began to entertain some hope of recovery. However, for that month of abandonment by the "hope of the elderly", HMO's, I was left with the opinion that some of them manage only money, not health care. I shall always feel that someone owes me for that often used phrase, pain and suffering.

Other things began to happen. Together Michelle and Karen shopped for food and stocked the refrigerator. They waited on me hand and foot, implementing the most important phase of recovery, that of staying off my feet and giving my hip a chance to improve.

They took turns, whichever one was here, keeping track of Dave. At one point God graciously provided thirteen consecutive days of April showers which narrowed Dave's arena of activity to inside the house and garage, a great blessing for us, a total bore for him.

When Karen had to return to her work, Michelle, although handicapped with a cast on a fractured elbow, came night after night to prepare supper with her one working hand, serving me with a tray on my lap. She would have done this much earlier if I, with my pride, had not kept my needs concealed from her. Dear Mullein Hill Church also responded with meals, as is typical of them.

During this time Dave had cataract surgery. With crutches in hand I managed to get him where he had to be for all his appointments. Driving was not a problem, though getting in and out of the car was an exhibition of creep, crawl, and complain. I was always thankful to arrive home to my chair.

Accompanying my return of hope was gratitude -- to God, and to family, for being there for me, even though I had lost sight of them all for a few days. The responsibilities of caring for Dave leave no time for me to be incapacitated. This primary learning experience was stark and scary, and from it came the sustaining assurance that there are those in my life who are there for me.

I feel compelled to share this episode in my life with others who may need permission to expose their real feelings when they have been plummeted into a similar abyss. God alone knows how human we are and surely is not surprised, nor does He judge us, when we slip into feelings of hopelessness and desolation. We seem to feel the need to deny those feelings to each other, and even to ourselves. They just don't feel very spiritual! We somehow have the compulsion to hide behind a benign victory attitude, the stiff upper lip and the brave smile, in order to present an image of trust and serenity that really isn't there at all. That is a phony facade and certainly does not serve others well.

I have been strengthened and cheered to find that occasionally even the giants of our faith have had their deep-down times of struggle and have had to reassess Whose they were. Just read the Psalms. I am encouraged by those who let me know of their anguish. Among other things it gives me permission to let others know when I have a struggle I cannot handle alone.

This crisis has taught me much. It has strengthened my faith. It has taught me that family is here. It has reminded me that we aren't going to do it my way. We will do it His way. It has told me again that no matter how I feel, He is always there, regardless of circumstances. I realize in a new way how very vulnerable we are and how easily we fall into unbelief, as did the father in Mark 9:24, whose son was afflicted with an evil spirit. Bill Gaither sings a heart-catching song, "I Believe. Help Thou My Unbelief." I play it over and over. Thank you, Bill Gaither, for touching that spot in my life.

In consideration of my humanness I know I have not learned, once and for all, all that I will have to learn about this subject as the days pass. Some of this ground I will undoubtedly have to weed and cultivate again and again. Weeds seem to be as prevalent in our lives and as demanding of our attention as they are in the garden.

But at least for now this plateau of Yankee independence has been thoroughly plowed, harrowed, and replanted. Allowing that fallow ground to be broken up was a hard lesson. I hope I will not have to relearn it too often.

Chapter 16

TREASURES

As I sat during those difficult days of sampling things which were entirely distasteful to me, such as learning to be somewhat more dependent on others, I was also aware of one more struggle. What was I to do with our earthly treasures?

I was not prepared for the intense feelings which accompanied my thoughts of parting with things, many of which had made our home distinctly ours. These were the things which we had given each other over the years, the things given to us by our children, and then the very special things passed down to us from other generations, especially my grandparents.

The latter group of treasures had played a very special role in the lives of my brother and me. Those grandparents had kept us from being victims of a broken home. Possessions of theirs which I am privileged to see every day are my constant reminders of their role in our lives. Consequently, when I found myself unable to cope physically with the demands of caring for a home, I was shaken thoroughly. Home was a place where not only were ones' children loved, nurtured, treasured, and prepared for moving on as a capable next generation; one also lived with things, and cared for them, and passed them on to that next generation.

This had been the practice in our family. Some of my dearest treasures belonged to those grandparents. Some even had been passed down from their parents.

I had never before found it necessary to address the subject of leaving those things behind. Nor would I have expected it to be a problem. Suddenly I found myself in a state of deep mourning. I felt inconsolable, almost as if being separated from those precious things was akin to someone dying.

I was already saying good-bye to my husband as he became more and more an impersonal stranger. Must I also say good-bye to those things which held such special memories for me?

It seemed I was the only one left to care. Not true, of course. Our children are now adults, have their own homes, and also have an attachment for those treasures. I knew all that, but something seemed to blot the reality from my mind.

Perhaps any thought of delegating our treasures indicated the end of an era. Was it the end of being in our own home? I can't explain how all the subjects got so intertwined: Dave's Alzheimer's, my disability, the possibility of leaving 14 Greenbrier Drive with its treasures after 22 years of it being our home. I guess the thought of being in that long-term care facility somewhere, forever sitting and waiting in those geri-chairs seemed to be more of a reality than ever. And all because I could not function adequately.

Was I feeling guilty and to blame? I don't know. What I do know is that I was feeling total turmoil, and at that point I could neither handle it, nor ignore it.

This impasse nudged me into considering my value system. My earthly treasures, all of a sudden, were no longer my joys. They had become spiritual liabilities.

Reason reminded me how earthbound we humans are, especially those of us who value the past and the people who made it special by their contributions to our lives. They leave many reminders behind that in a sense tie us to our past.

I looked at my Nana's silver, her pewter which she had acquired through an old mail-order chain called "Larkin's", some of her china, her fern stand...

Grampa's favorite silver spoon with its bowl broken nearly off its handle from use for nearly 80 years still gives me a sense of warm nostalgia each time I polish it and place it back in its slot on my spoon rack. I remember setting the table for Nana and always placing Grampa's special spoon by his knife even though it didn't match anything else.

His collar box, with his shirt studs and ruby-studded gold cuff links adorn my bureau. What to do with those? No one else had the memories of helping him put his celluloid collar on with those studs as I had done when I was a child. His old hands had eventually become unable to handle such small things.

These were just a few of my precious possessions, but I knew as I pondered this whole subject that I had things quite out of focus. My real focus should be Heaven. Those material things which I had inherited and adored had to be of less importance than the inheritance which I knew was waiting for me in Heaven, the focal point of which was Jesus Himself. Instead, I was very aware that Heaven seemed to be playing second-fiddle.

I did some careful evaluating about a new subject in my life, that of icons and idols. My friend Webster says an idol is "a representation to which worship is addressed." I quickly ruled out idols. My theology was too good for that. But what about icons? An icon is "a representation of a venerated person," so says Webster. Hmmm. There was nothing wrong with venerating the memory of my grandparents, but to let their representation become so important -- there certainly was something wrong with that.

I shared my feelings with my brother. He understood. He told me of his own struggle in resolving this same quandary. His attachment had been best handled by deciding to revere those things, along with their precious memories, for as long as he lived and could do so. After that, the real people would again be a part of his life because they had come to know Jesus in their 80's and there was Eternity to share with them. Their old things down here would matter little.

How I needed that point of view! I thank my brother for his input. As I pondered it, my focus began to clear.

A talk with our daughters further cleared my head. "Just put our names on the things you'd like us to have," they said. "They are important to us, too." "And why haven't you told us you were feeling so troubled," one daughter asked. I had no answer.

Circumstances did not change but my attitude did, and I began to see why I had reacted so strongly. Too much happening at once. Too much to try to handle alone. Too much thinking all by myself and feeling so keenly the loss of the other half of me who normally would be part of the solution. Plus an enormous sense of guilt because I couldn't just make all the problems go away. Isn't that what mothers do? Make everything O.K? Like taking our child with the injured ant she held so tenderly in her grubby little hand and helping her place it back where she had found it so its mother would come and make it all better. Only this time that wouldn't work.

Overload? Perhaps. That's what we label lots of things today. And part of my overload was realizing afresh how much is lost when two people who have shared lives, things, and thoughts for over 55 years are denied that privilege for the remainder of their time together. The undertaking for the one who finds himself in charge can be ponderous and unwieldy.

What I hadn't remembered was the fact that nothing is overload for my Father. Strange how I keep having trouble with things I was so sure I knew all about.

Chapter 17

ONLY ON LOAN

While I was agonizing over the possibility of having to relinquish those personal elements which help us make our lives on this planet uniquely ours, little did I realize that God indeed had an important lesson for me. That lesson is one I would have confidently and somewhat defensively protested I knew all about.

But I didn't know all about it, and when I learned it, it led to the end of the struggles that had dominated the last four months of my life. It opened up to me a totally unexpected and completely satisfying resting place.

That release came by way of a Gaither video on which Gloria Gaither recalled the words of a song:

"May I always remember the things dear to my heart

Are mine to hold only by the Grace of God."

Those two lines caused me to become aware, down deep in my very being, that everything any of us has,

EVERYTHING, each other, our precious children, health, home, treasures, *everything*, is after all only on loan to us. The realization swept over me like a refreshing and restoring breeze.

May I repeat, I was sure I knew all that. But as can happen to all humans, under the pressure of difficult circumstances I surely lost sight of it. Perhaps I had never dealt in depth with this truth I knew, because when the test came Satan insidiously stole my victory.

Only on loan! How I needed that release. I was no longer hostage to anything in my life, as I surely had been. It doesn't mean that I value people and things less. I just hold them more loosely, and I bask in the knowledge that God, in His singular and personal way, has seen fit to let me have them to enjoy for a time -- His time. Such liberation. My heart sang.

Since that day I have had quietness and peace of mind over all that had caused me such anguish. I thank the Gaithers for a ministry that meets us right where we are living at the moment. They remind us of the truths of our Faith with such simplicity and joy.

With enthusiasm I shared this wonderful on loan reality with Dave and felt disappointment that he was not able to understand. The family did, however, to my joy and deep satisfaction.

Some days later I found Dave sitting in his chair, eyes closed, face drawn and sad. I inquired gently why he looked so very sad, and he responded, "I'm having such a terrible time coping with the loss of my mind. I used to have a brain."

I always felt entirely inadequate to comfort him when this wave of mourning descended upon him, as it often did.

This time my lights flashed on. Only on loan! Perhaps he could grasp that concept as it applied to his own circumstance. So while trying not to sound preachy I reminded him gently of all the years he had used that fine mind which God had given him to carefully teach the Word. Dave had regarded that mind as his most precious asset. I reminded him that it had been on loan to him for over 80 years. I suggested that if God now saw fit to take any part of it back, perhaps he could formally give God permission to do so.

His immediate reply was, "How would I do that?" I suggested that as he had urged his people over the years to just talk to God about their problems, he could do the same. His favorite verse for years had been, "Call unto me and I will answer thee, and show thee great and mighty things which thou knowest not." (Jer. 33:3 KJV) I suggested he call upon the promise of that verse just now, once again in his life.

We bowed our heads. He prayed. He prayed a lovely prayer: family, friends, church, missionaries, etc., and said his Amen. No mention of the real subject.

I praised his beautiful prayer, but suggested gently that he had not addressed his real subject. He looked surprised. "I didn't?", he asked.

I suggested he try again. Same sort of prayer. He did not remember what he had said previously.

Again I reminded him of his subject. He tried once more, and this time he addressed, head on, his real subject. I had the feeling that the first two attempts were his way of priming the pump in order to start the flow of something he hardly dared to voice.

He expressed his gratitude for the mind which had been entrusted to him. He was able to tell God that he was giving back what was now left; he gave his permission for God to do with the remainder whatever He saw fit. It was a direct sincere encounter, and for Dave, a difficult one.

We shared tears and some commune time until he regained his composure.

Since that day he has not once said, "I used to have a brain," a comment he had made often during recent years. And while the sadness is still there at times, he appears to have a peace which has not been evident for a long time.

I am neither a songwriter, nor a poet, but it seems to me someone must write a song with lyrics saying:

> *Not mine to own, not mine to keep*
> *Here are my treasures, Lord*
> *I leave them at your feet.*
> *Not mine to own, only on loan*
> *Keep me remembering*
> *That they are yours alone.*

Or something like that.

Gwen Bibber Kimball

Chapter 18

GARDENS

As Dave and I stroll, trudge or stumble our way along, whichever pace fits the events of the day, one subject brings more pain to me than most others. It is a subject I had overlooked when I so casually used the word "everything" in regard to my treasures. That is the subject of my gardens. The struggle surrounding them presented me with one of my greatest conflicts, a conflict I did not handle well.

For years, as we left home after home and yard after yard, things were always far more attractive when we left than when we came. I sadly stroked my evergreens, shrubs and flowers good-bye many times.

Now we have a yard which has been put together over a 20-year period in company with daughter, Michelle, and which looks like a small park in the spring. Our profusion of rhododendrons and azaleas bloom from mid-April 'til mid-July. Our dogwoods produce those long awaited splashes of color after a long winter.

A lovely Japanese thread-leaf maple is among the prizes, along with a mountain laurel and a weeping cherry, all gifts from family and friends on special occasions like birthdays, mother's day, etc.

We have an assortment of ferns, and wild flowers which hardly anyone grows these days such as jack-in-the-pulpits, painted trilliums, princess pine, bunchberries, ladies' slippers, yellow, blue, and white violets and partridgeberries, to name a few. I handle these all with tender care, and rejoice each spring when they begin to make an appearance.

Funniest thing. Dave, who never was a gardener, hardly knew there was a garden except to exclaim over how beautiful everything was and how proud he was of it all; never saw a weed, nor would he have known one if he did see it; he added these gardens to his picking up fervor. It became an absolute obsession, every twig, every day that weather permitted. Pick up, pick up, tramp, tramp, numberless times a day all through these growing things, just to retrieve his little twigs he saw everywhere. Can you imagine what his size nine shoes and his 180+ pounds were doing, not only to plants, but to soil and root systems? And can you imagine what Dave's very size was doing to branches of shrubs?

Yet, if I suggested to him however gently that I'd take care of the gardens as I always had done, he considered it an "absolute affront, and a denying of his rights to go where he wanted on HIS property." "After all," he would remind me, "that yard is as much mine as yours." The subject had nothing to do with forgetting. It was his determined decision that the gardens were his to do with as he liked. Again, welcome to the Alzheimer's world, I told myself.

Yet, I don't know if this unreasonable attitude was all just Alzheimer's, or if it had something to do with Grandmother telling him what to do. Perhaps it went back to the subject of losing control as head of his home.

At any rate, after much reminding, pleading, coaxing and even scolding, I found myself reduced to pure fury. On the one hand I was then trying to justify all that fury, and on the other hand I was not liking myself very much because of it.

But these gardens were like my children I was trying to defend! And they represented the last personal area I had left. Almost all other aspects of my life were swallowed up by one single consideration. That one consideration which totally swamped my entire life, I told myself petulantly, was ALZHEIMER'S. I even have to say good-bye to my gardens! Not a noble attitude, but occasionally a typical one for caregivers, I'm sure.

I told myself there had to be a way to work this out and still have the gardens. Occasionally Dave would relent and promise he would not go in them, ever again, and he even wrote a pledge and signed it! Next day, in his Alzheimer's world he was back to the gardens again.

The solution? I finally came to a conclusion. It was hard, tearfully hard. It took courage. I had to add my gardens to my earlier decision regarding all my treasures. They must join the ranks of not mine to own, only on loan. They must be included in the EVERYTHING. I would say no more.

With that decision my emotions seemed to settle into a flat calm for the next three or four days. I steadfastly ignored what was going on outside and told myself I didn't care. Denial, perhaps?

Those days of calm left me totally unprepared for the next set of emotions, those of a warm and sickly-cozy feeling of martyrdom. It felt so good, and I felt so gratifyingly sorry for myself. What is it about becoming a martyr to a cause that envelops one in a sort of cloak of false solace, almost like a self-patronizing ego trip. Whatever it was, I was in it.

However, not being a martyr at heart, I put an end to that phase quite promptly, and found it being replaced by my old fury again. This time I was furious at being trapped. I could not safeguard my gardens, I could not go on being a martyr, and I could not be angry the remainder of our lives. My feelings that "if Dave only cared enough, etc., etc.," were unrealistic because I knew he did care, but his mind could no longer handle those concepts. "Of course I care," he repeatedly reassured me, as he strode through the plants. I was trapped, for sure.

My only recourse? Accept reality and let them go, let them go, again and again, and perhaps cope with the same emotions, again and again. I could not go on being hostage to my gardens at the cost of constant turmoil and unpleasantness. *Not mine to own, only on loan.*

I put forth a profound effort. As time passed I found I did have a few relapses, and on occasion I did entertain some of those old martyrdom feelings, but for the most part I was able to let them go. The fact that the ground was frozen and many of the plants were away for the winter helped me to ignore the many forays during those less crucial months.

What I could not foresee was an event out ahead of us which would put those gardens, once and for all, into their proper perspective, and after which, with deep peace in my heart, I would never feel any desire to mention them to Dave again.

Chapter 19

HEARING AIDS

This chapter is written with tongue in cheek and I would invite you to assume the same pose, should you care to. I must indulge my Irish genes as I comment on another issue which we really didn't need to have as a companion to Alzheimer's, that of Dave's deafness.

Deafness is aided in this space age by a terribly flawed (my opinion) device known as a hearing aid. This little-noticed agent, worn discreetly in the ear, provides a somewhat less that perfect assist to the listener. I am informed that the tonal qualities leave much to be desired.

It breaks easily, especially in the hands of a one-time marine machinist who hasn't exactly spent his latter years doing fancy work. Dave does most things with a heavy touch, such as, when he gives me a pat I have to remind him that I am not a horse.

This device runs on tiny batteries that defy the manual skills of hands the size of a lady's, much less those of a man.

It takes delight in running out of steam during church, or some such interesting place. On unpredictable occasions it enjoys singing when it should be just listening, such as in restaurants when the wearer adds the simple stimulus of setting his jaws in motion in order to chew his dinner.

For the communicator it provides an opportunity for a considerable erosion of patience. I sometimes complain/explain to God that this entire Alzheimer's journey would be ever so much easier if only Dave weren't deaf. Nearly everything I say in life I say at least twice, many things three or more times, causing me to intone silently in the back of my head, "ONE MORE TIME!" (Not one of my more praiseworthy attitudes). At least, Dave never knows.

Words that get past the hearing aids not only have to be repeated, they sometimes have to be spelled, and then they often have to be explained. Of course, even then they still may not penetrate through to that mysteriously lost ability to comprehend.

Dave wore two aids for a while, but the expense of keeping two of them repaired reduced us to one. Just one provides adequate budget damage.

Then there is the constantly recurring problem of, "What did I do with it?" We have spent endless hours searching, and have found it in the most innovative places. Once it was found between pages in the telephone book. Who would ever think to look there, especially when the wearer can't hear enough to use the phone in the first place? It was found purely by chance, but with great joy and rejoicing, after being missing for too many days.

I am reminded of another lost hearing aid event which lasted for nearly two weeks. Picture the search. In his bed, in every drawer, in every closet, in the washer, in the drier, under every piece of furniture, under every cushion, among all the books in our several book areas, in the car, in the garage, around the yard, around the work bench, in the vacuum cleaner bag, in all Dave's pockets, etc., etc. Each day we repeated the effort. It had to be somewhere, didn't it? At that point, I was beginning to wonder.

Throughout our search Dave would slip into that typical fog which so obscures the real world of these victims, and he would ask in total blandness, "What in the world are we doing?" "We are looking for your hearing aid, Dear." "Oh." The search would continue, punctuated by the same question at regular intervals. And on, and on.

Finally we gave up. It seemed that our only option was to buy another for better than half a thousand dollars. Karen predicted that one day Dad would come strolling out complete with hearing aid in his ear with no memory of having lost it, and with no idea where he had found it, so we waited a bit...

Sure enough, out of the blue one morning out walked Dave with his hearing aid in its proper place. I exclaimed with much enthusiasm, "Oh, you found your hearing aid. Where in the world was it?" With a look of mild surprise Dave replied, "Oh, was it lost?"

I foolishly wasted both his time and mine by attempting to remind him of our long and fruitless search, and of course he remembered not a minute of it, nor could he remember where he had just found it. "Beats me," was his only comment. My silent response was, "Duh!!!!" as I mentally bumped my forehead with the palm of my hand and intoned again (to myself), "Welcome to Alzheimer's."

It even went through the wash once, which of course did it in. Memory of the repair bill is a constant reminder to check pockets on laundry day.

With the loss of some of his normal manual dexterity Dave drops it occasionally, which can also result in a trip to the repair shop. Every time it is there, of course, we live with the added frustration of his not hearing even as much (or as little) as he does with it.

Another side of the hearing aid dilemma is Dave's inability to realize whether or not the battery is working. If it isn't, then he is wearing a very effective earplug! So we go through the routine of, "Do you have your hearing aid in, Dear?" The answer to that is always, "Yes." If not, we find it. Next step: "Is it turned up?" The answer to that is always, "Yes," also. So we go through a check to make sure. If it is not turned up, we again go through the routine of, "Turn it up 'til it squeals, and then turn it back slightly, Dear." This cycle is necessary every single time, without fail.

If the battery is dead I go to my hiding place, a spot known only to me. Too many times we ran out of batteries without my knowing. I was finding little batteries around here and there, always asking, "Are these used or new?" "Beats me." Easier to keep track of such matters myself, even though it is one more thing. Imagine the days when he wore two very effective earplugs.

I am now realizing that there is a conflict for Dave between hearing and understanding. His inability to process information well may account partially for what seems to be inability to hear. What he does hear he hears more slowly than formerly. Even his hour of news, morning and evening, which has been of prime importance for years, now moves too fast for him to assimilate.

His common comment is, "Do you know what in the world they're talking about?" He no longer understands that I have not yet mastered the skill of listening and talking at the same time, and that if I try to tell him what he has just missed, I am missing what is just now being said. All he is able to gather is that he can't understand any of it, and I am not being any help. He very often leaves the room before the news is over.

Add to that the universal habit of the hard-of-hearing person to automatically say "What?" the first time around, and then commence listening the second time around. I am trying to learn to face Dave, get his attention, and then articulate carefully and slowly. However, it goes without saying that this is not always a convenient procedure to follow when driving. Facing your passenger long enough to say something could facilitate one problem and cause another!

One must remember, too, that just about every subject is new every time it comes up, as if it had never come up before. Two of Dave's favorite comments are, "News to me", and, "You could fool me." I hear both on a regular basis. Usually those responses don't bother me, but sometimes I exhibit a classic example of Philip Yancey's wonderful word, "ungrace" as I walk away intoning to myself (with a smile on my face!), "So what else is new." This type of response doesn't occur too often, and when it does I don't feel especially virtuous. But an understanding Father thankfully knows about limits, and doesn't demand a perfect score. He permits me lapses in grace because He above all others knows all about my humanness. I am thankful for that, and of course my brief moment of impropriety presents me with one of these rare occasions when I am thankful that Dave can't hear!

One evening in the car I realized I was nearly shouting as Dave and I tried to converse. I finally said, "Honey, is your hearing aid working?" Care to guess his answer? Of course, it was "Yes." "Well, why don't we just check it anyway?" Through the routine of turn it up, etc., sure enough, the battery was dead. "Let me put it in my purse for safekeeping," I said. Dave's solution? "I'd rather keep it in my ear so I'll know where it is." No realization that in so doing he was inserting that very effective earplug, again.

We eventually returned to two aids: two earplugs, two to find, two to check for dead batteries, two to regulate for volume. (At least, when you find one you find the other, usually).

It was pointed out to me one weekend, very kindly and gently, that in my weariness and frustration over handling life for two, and of having to repeat continually, my voice eventually takes on a demeaning quality. I do not want that to happen. Dave cannot help either his deafness or his illness. I appreciated being told, and while I assume I do not always avoid it, I am now conscious of how I sound in a new way. Most of the time I am glad for the chance to care for my Dear One, hearing aids and all, and I try desperately hard to do so with grace and patience.

Please don't casually put this subject aside as too small a thing to write about in a book. Believe me! It is just one more contributor to the 36-hour-day of the caregiver. When I have a day or two off one of the most obvious contributors to the change is *not having to repeat.*

However, as I conclude that God has trusted me with Dave's Alzheimer's, I conclude also that He has trusted me with his deafness. I at times deplore and seriously question His confidence in me.

And if by chance you did read this with tongue in cheek, may we now all return to normal and go on to another subject.

Chapter 20

TUNING OUT

Right or wrong, cop-out or reality, a matter of sheer pique or an attempt at survival? I am still in the process of deciding. Perhaps it is a little of each. This concerns my involuntary and mechanical reaction to certain of Dave's episodes of rage when they become directed at me. In spite of my firm conviction that his attitudes and responses are part of an illness, there is a threshold, the crossing of which, on occasion, propels me into a vacuum of "no feel."

I find myself totally tuning out, making no eye contact, feeling a-emotional, and moving about as if in a solitary world, almost as though Dave did not exist in this very same room with me. I shut my emotional doors, close my blinds, and pretend I am not at home to anyone except myself.

It seems I need to do this while I stop hurting; I need to do this until I can handle Dave's out-of-control behavior and the resulting personal onslaughts that are hurled in my direction; I need to do this until I can again handle reality. I also need to regard these feelings as legitimate for this place in time, because they seem to provide me with survival time until I can find the switch that resets my focus on his illness instead of on my woundedness.

As yet, I have not found that switch that allows me to do this instantaneously. I seem to have to dwell for a time on inwardly viewing Dave as an ingrate for whom I am giving my life, nearly every waking hour; for whom nearly every decision is made, and for whom nearly every consideration is first taken into account. How dare he be this way! How dare he call me names and shout at me. MY personhood is also important, I tell myself loftily, in my walled-off solitary spot; let's see how he gets along without me and my care; he'll end up wishing he had chosen to be courteous and gentlemanly when he finds out how much he needs me -- and on -- and on.

The process of defending myself and my own dignity FEELS SO GOOD! For a while I thoroughly enjoy it. My silent message is, "Don't try to reach me. I'm not here. I've left, and I just may not come back."

Recovery times vary, but eventually the obvious reappears. These episodes are Dave's response to his need to lash out in protest against his awful circumstances, and I am the nearest target. It is not personal in any way.

Why does it seem so personal to me sometimes? I think "saturation" has something to do with it. Just as too much rain cannot run off fast enough to prevent an overload of water upon the landscape, the human spirit can absorb just so much, emotionally, without the same normal consequence. The flood of emotions has to have time to abate. At least this becomes my rationale for the response I make to those events in my life which I am learning to handle.

My self-exile is usually short-lived. I presently open my doors and blinds, recognize that there are two of us in this home, and go about admitting Dave back into my life as a valued and full-fledged part of me.

Meanwhile, he has ceased being angry, doesn't even know he was, and wouldn't believe his behavior if I told him. He responds to a hug and a pat, though he is totally unaware that I have just punished him by making him an outcast. For this I am thankful. He does not need isolation added to his list of burdens.

I presume I will tune out on numerous occasions in the future, but experience tells me that it will come to a fairly speedy conclusion each time. Meanwhile, I will have gained recovery time, and it will be my secret, because dear, dear Dave Kimball need never know that for a very brief time I went away.

Gwen Bibber Kimball

Chapter 21

SAMANTHA

And then there is Samantha. Samantha is our very special kitty, not a cat, please! Any feline can be called a cat. Samantha is not to be so designated because she is not just any feline. And Kitty does not mean kitten. At nearly 20 years of age she would hardly fit that designation. She is our kitty: arrogant, demanding, independent, and decidedly aloof. She is completely capable of asserting her silent opinion of things by her superb body language. She manages all of us. Even Dave Kimball. Tunnel-visioned, dedicated dog lover that he is, he condescends to scratch her ears and tell her, "You're a good kid," though I suspect he feels patronized that she even permits it.

When she decides to do so she humors us with her attention, sings us lovely songs, cuddles up to get rockied (baby talk for rocked, as in a rocking chair). When she comes in from the cold she agrees to having her trotters (more baby talk meaning feet) held in a warm hand until she decides *that's enough of that.*

These affectations are somewhat recent ones for Samantha. When she came to us somewhere in 1980-81 she was apparently looking for a better place to eat, sleep, and catch birds. We heard a pitiful crying one rainy night outside a basement window and there stood this wet, dirty little animal which we of course recognized as a cat. But we were not in the market for a cat, so we ignored It so It would look further. It apparently liked what It saw and decided to hang around a bit longer. Consequently It was still there the next evening.

My grandmother-heart became an easy touch and I proffered a small saucer of milk. After all, "the poor little thing, etc., etc., and It *is* kind of pretty." Everything changed. It stayed. It ate, and ate. It started washing up, and a beautiful animal began to emerge. On good authority we were told It was a Himalayan. That means part Persian, part Siamese; silky buff-colored coat, long brown fluffy tail, seal-point ears, boots on Its feet, gorgeous blue eyes, and the crowning feature of a huge white ruff around Its neck.

We decided on a visit to the vet who pronounced It to be a she who had recently had a litter of kittens, was probably a year and a half old or so, and would make a lovely pet.

Michelle had immediately become Its mother, and along with other family members started pleading, "Oh, keep her," which caused us all to feel indicted and convicted of something dreadful if we decided otherwise.

By now we were totally trapped, so we fell willingly in line as grandmother, grandfather, and aunties, none of us feeling that we had violated those roles by including a kitty in the family circle. However, in deference to those who object to the designations we will eliminate capital letters.

We had her spayed. In came food and a litter box. We then instituted a formal search for a name appropriate to this lovely creature who by now was being treated as if she were our very first child. How is it that cats, excuse me, kitties, can do that to intelligent humans?

According to the vet, this cat who had become our kitty almost overnight had not been treated very well; she had a broken tooth which he said was unusual, and to him indicated the possibility of abuse. Indeed, her behavior showed a considerable lack of confidence in people. Any move toward her, or even the extension of a hand in her direction caused her to duck out of reach. Her reactions were decidedly spooky. Samantha, of "Bewitched," TV fame, seemed to be the obvious role model in our attempt to select a name, and that choice has been confirmed over and over again. Consequently, It became Samantha, Sammie for short.

The living-in process went nicely as long as we honored Samantha's wishes. We learned early on that if it wasn't Sammie's idea, forget it, no matter how well intentioned your thought was. However, that thought would probably become her thought about the time you'd given up on it, all of this being in strict cat tradition, of course.

During this process of adoption I found out why my grandmother would not have a cat when we children lived at the Lake with her. She always said it was because of her lovely birds. Childlike, I didn't think there was any contest between birds and cats. Anyone should know you couldn't play with birds. Anyway, we had no cat at the Lake and after Sammie had been with us for a short time I knew why. The poor birds that frequented our feeder didn't stand a chance. Sammie would even take down Blue-jays. The feeder was quite promptly retired to a back corner of our garage, but it was a long time before those angry birds stopped stalking Sammie whenever she was outside. They even sat on the gutters and looked for her inside the windows, all the while screaming unintelligible but obviously very naughty things at her.

The ravages of time are quite evident with Sammie these days. She and I are both exhibiting signs of lameness by adopting the gait of penguins, and we often commiserate with each other when our hips and legs hurt and we both sort of stagger around the house. She apparently no longer sees too well either, and I suspect her hearing is about gone. Her once soft gentle cry is now a totally disruptive caterwaul, repeated nine or ten times in succession, as if the whole world couldn't have heard it the first time. Several people have come completely off their chairs, and one friend's prayer time was abruptly terminated with, "Amen! and what was THAT?"

Samantha has spent her later years sleeping and eating. She does wash her face and hands after eating, but she is not able to groom herself anymore. Her lovely coat which once glistened is now somewhat matted and lusterless, in spite of attempts at keeping her combed. But in her retirement years there is an added element: she has become my confidant. She now asks to sit in my lap, and as communication slowly fails with Grandfather, I talk things over with Sammie. She is a good listener, responds to me by cuddling on my shoulder, finding a special song to sing and rubbing my hand with her chin, and she doesn't panic if I cry a bit.

Her bedtime routine remains intact. She lets me know it's time for me to turn out the lights and go to bed by sitting by my chair and caterwauling. She can no longer jump up by herself, so I carry her in and place her on the bed. When I am finished with my bedtime reading I turn out my bedside light, cuddle her up to me, stroke her while she sings me a little song and has a nap. However, when that nap is over she makes it evident that that's it. I put her down and she goes out to her favorite spot, directly in front of a heat vent where she spends most of her time letting the warmth comfort her old bones.

Someday she will not be there for that little bedtime routine and I shall miss it sorely, just as I shall miss the rockies and other moments we have shared. I shall miss her indulgence in permitting me to whisper some of my private thoughts in her ear, and her tolerance for my telling her repeatedly how special she is. Most of all I shall always think of her companionship whenever I sit alone by the fireside in the evening. I can't imagine her not being there.

Addendum, June 8, 1999

Our lovely Samantha was put to sleep today. She was deteriorating with her advanced years, and the only reason to keep her any longer would be my own selfishness. So I called the vet, made the appointment, and then watched the hours pass. A few minutes before getting out her kitty wagon I held her for a last rocky, and she sang me a quiet little song, but I also discovered that she had become incontinent, a fact which helped verify to me that this was the right time. It helped diminish my grief.

She showed little resistance to her ride, and except for the pinch of the shot, to which she objected aggressively, she went to sleep peacefully as we stroked her and loved her through her time of final good-bye. And even though Dave's name for Sammie for years had been "Jug-head" and I had not expected him to go into any great emotional spasm over her passing, he did exhibit a sadness which I found to be surprising and gratifying.

Instead of cremation as we had planned, we dug deep into a shady flower bed for a spot to lay her. We wrapped her in a pink pillowcase, filtered the soil gently over the still warm and pliable little form, intermingling the soil with our good-byes. We laid a slate stone over "her place," and topped it with a flowering potted plant.

This morning her absence was obvious, but I stepped to the window and called, "Good morning, Dolly," to her. Somehow Sammie's place in my heart is still full, though in a way, empty, but I am satisfied. And come to think of it, she, like everything and everyone else in our lives, was only on loan from God for a time, anyway.

Chapter 22

MARTHA'S VINEYARD

The day dawned foggy and gray in New Bedford -- not an unusual start for those of us who are privileged to live on the seacoast. It looked as if our plans for a day trip by the ferry *Schamonchi* to Martha's Vineyard were about to be put on hold.

That would be a disappointment to Karen, Michelle, and me, (if not for Dave who disavowed any tolerance for anything which took him from the comfort of his Lazyboy lounger). We had approached this day with great anticipation. For several years it had been our privilege to sail the Maine Coast on the Windjammer, the *Mary Day* out of Camden with Capt. Havilah S. Hawkins, who had become a much loved part of our family. Now his son Havilah, better known as "Haddie" was sailing his own vessel, the *Vela* out of Martha's Vineyard, one of those Island jewels off the Massachusetts coast.

We had made our plans with Haddie but now we pondered if we wanted to spend good money just to look into a fog bank at Martha's Vineyard, when we could do that at home for free!

A call to the weather bureau assured us that indeed the sun was shining on the Vineyard so, complete with lunch, binoculars, sun glasses, etc., we drove to the ferry parking lot, left the car and boarded the ferry.

We agreed that Dave could not wander too far on the ferry, or get into too much trouble, so we kept an eye open but left him free to explore on his own, for most of the one hour trip, indulging him with a cup of coffee and a goodie on the way. That kept him seated in one spot and we knew just where he was for at least part of the time!

Michelle, Karen and I stood at the bow and watched our progress as we passed through Wood's Hole -- a Navigator's challenge even in clear weather, and sure enough, we came out into full sunshine as we approached the village of Vineyard Haven, our port on Martha's Vineyard. We found Haddie waiting for us on the beach with his yawl boat, and a short row took us to his very pretty *Vela* moored a short distance off shore.

We spent the day on the water, a number 10 day to sail. Warm sun, a steady breeze, and plenty of time to catch up on days gone by with Capt. Haddie, and his wife Beverly who was our most gracious hostess.

Dave was perhaps a bit less enthusiastic. "Sailing is O.K.," he would comment, "but all the seats are so hard." Even the addition of cushions didn't convince him otherwise. But he adjusted graciously and really came alive when Beverly emerged from the galley with a lovely tray of hors d'oeuvres. As the tray reached Dave he lost track of reality and decided that this was his lunch! We managed to head that idea off without undue embarrassment for him, and whether he understood or not, the tray survived many rounds without further incident. That was our only problem during our several hours of enjoying the beautiful waters of Nantucket Sound.

We came ashore at the town of Edgartown and boarded a bus for a short run back to Vineyard Haven and our ferry, for our return trip to New Bedford. Dave couldn't understand why we were on a bus. "Why don't we just use our car?", he asked. "Because it is back on the mainland," we replied. "We have to take the ferry to get back there". He remained bewildered about it and much discussion did not convince him. As we approached the ferry landing he was sure that wasn't even our ferry, but he acquiesced and boarded with us, and we breathed a sigh of relief. We had him where he needed to be to make our way home, and with our relief there was a measure of complacency.

After boarding, Dave went on a tour. He had done well on the trip over, so what harm? The ferry backed away from the landing, headed out of the harbor, and suddenly we heard the loud speaker crackle on with an announcement: "The Captain has been informed that there is a family aboard who are on the wrong ferry and need to be let off, so we are in the process of returning to the dock." We three sat quietly and waited for this poor misdirected family to emerge and leave the ferry.

About the same time Karen said, "By the way, I wonder where Dad is." She strolled off on a search. and when she found him she said, "Oh, here you are! What have you been doing?", never dreaming what she was about to hear. "Oh, I've been up to the bridge to let the Captain know that we shouldn't be on this ferry!", he said, with some agitation. He had obviously been quite eloquent and convincing, considering the announcement we had just heard all over the ship! The Captain must have felt he had no reason to question the word of this fine appearing gentleman.

Karen arrived back with her dad, and seeming somewhat disconcerted she said, "Here's Dad. I've got to go."

She went immediately to the bridge. "Did a gentleman come up here and tell you a family was on the wrong ferry?", she asked. "Yes," replied the Captain. Karen began a litany of apologies which seemed not to impress Sir Captain. My dad has Alzheimer's," she explained, "and we lost track of him for a few minutes. I am *so* sorry." After much abject apologizing Karen arrived back with the family unit where we finally found out what had actually transpired, and how involved our dad had really been!

"I'll give the Captain the benefit of the doubt," Karen said. "Perhaps he's just phlegmatic by nature, but I never did so much bowing, scraping, and apologizing in my life as I did to that Captain!"

Meanwhile, Sir Captain had aborted the turn around and the ferry was again heading out of the harbor and home. We had an uneventful and pleasant trip, Dave's doubts as to our destination notwithstanding. As we de-barked in New Bedford Karen went again to the bridge to issue a final apology, and we did an encore of the bowing, the scraping, and the thank-yous toward the Captain's presence on the bridge. Dave, of course, had not a single clue as to what that was all about!

And how our car got there in that parking lot was a total mystery to Dave, but there it was! "Beats me," he said, he who also had no memory of our having left it there, of the trip in the fog that morning, or of our hours on the lovely *Vela*. He was satisfied to be heading home to the comfort of his Lazyboy, and we three were left with the poignant memories of our pristine day on the water with Haddie and Beverly, and of our latest Alzheimer's drama being enacted before an audience of 100 or so passengers.

Chapter 23

RESPITE

For the caregiver, life boils down to exactly one major word: TRAPPED. All 36 hours of every day, trapped. It doesn't even let up during the night. From it, there emerges another all-important word and that word is RESPITE.

Respite. Some hours off; a day or two now and then; or maybe even a week! No watching. No repeating. No need to know the where, the what, or the when of Dave's activities. The intervals that kept me from burn-out were those times when family and friends saw to it that I had a chance to leave it all, and have a change of pace and scenery.

Michelle asked me one day if I had written about this very important word. I hadn't. I decided to define and enlarge upon the word, so I sort of picked it apart with the help of my thesaurus. Respite implies an intermission, an interruption, a release, a parenthesis, a suspension, words which are all related to this trapped situation in their own singular way. Perhaps it is necessary to live in the environment of the victim in order to understand their full import as they relate to this trap, but as a substitute we will at least take a look.

This trap is inescapable and exhausting. There is never a letup, never a reprieve. It is just a way of life that becomes so routine and so habitual that it almost gets to seem normal, until all of a sudden someone says, "Isn't it time you had a day or two off?" And suddenly you think to yourself, "Oh, is there another life out there? I've forgotten."

Imagine getting into the car and driving away, all by yourself, knowing you haven't a care in the world for two whole days! I remember the first of many times that I did that. I took a deep breath and said out loud to myself, "Imagine, not one thing to think about!" It seemed like a fairy tale, and I kept repeating it to myself as if that would safeguard the event. Driving away by myself. What a novelty! No watching, no repeating...

The unthinkable part is that I never would have expected to feel that I had to escape from Dave Kimball. Here again is the need to keep the victim separate from the illness, even though this person may now bear only a slight resemblance to the one you hold in your memory.

As I consider this word, respite, I must pay tribute to the people who made it possible for me to put my things in the car and just leave, because that is what I did, and that is exactly how it felt. I just left.

Who made it possible? Chiefly, it was Michelle. A weekend with Karen at her home, or on a short flight somewhere, perhaps to hear the Gaither's, was a possibility only because of Michelle. She handled Dave well, and I had no worries while she was here. However, someone had to be with him until Michelle was home from her work day.

Enter Claire, faithful and dear, to take Dave for coffee, or to sit with him, or take him home to her house. Dave adored Claire, and supper with Claire and Michelle later on was a real treat for him.

In the earlier days, if Dave and Claire went out for coffee, Dave was always careful to be proper and let people know that, "My wife is away and my friend is treating me."

Claire always accommodated his nap time, either at home or at her house, and Dave always felt safe and cared for when with her. Many of my times away would have been impossible except for this very kind and caring friend.

Michelle spent many Saturdays and Sundays with Dave so I could be gone. Filling the hours with appropriate activities was no easy task and she did so with never a complaint.

Some Saturdays, she or Karen took Dave for the day, or for a few hours of the day, giving me a chance to enjoy the novelty of being alone in the house, and of being able to center my attention on some of my own interests.

Midgie lived too far away to be here often, but on occasionally she came so I could be gone for a week. Among those trips were one to Florida with dear Mrs. Ferrin, wife of the former President of Providence Bible Institute where Dave and I met; and another to the Grand Canyon with Karen, where we actually went rafting on the Colorado River!

Those times constituted a substantial enough break in routine that I almost felt disconnected from the reality that constituted "home." It felt so very far away. But the interlude was invaluable to my emotional survival, and I was always grateful that I could feel at peace with our arrangements for Dave.

Arriving home presented me with two feelings. One was of continuing on where I had left off, and the other was that of a whole new fresh beginning. Reality found me somewhere in between the two, but always benefiting from the change.

The professionals in my life kept reminding me of the danger of burnout and they were wise to do so. It is possible to become so involved in what seems to be a solitary responsibility that recognition of the need for relief and change escape you. That is especially so for people who tend to be independent.

There were times when only the people closest to me knew that it was time I had a break. I am forever indebted to them for their perception, and for standing in the gap to make breaks possible. "We are a family, and this is how it's done, Mom," they reminded me over and over. All I could do was shake my head, hug them, and reply, "Thank you for being here." The kind attention these special people provided just for *me* was of inestimable value. I could not have had it without them.

Gwen Bibber Kimball

Chapter 24

A MIND IN DISARRAY

As I write these pages, I am attempting to convey further features of this Alzheimer's landscape in which Dave and I live, move, and have our being.

I assume an artist scans his nearly finished piece of work and adds details in order to more fully clarify and complete that which he is wishing to portray. So it is, here.

Particulars come to mind as I read our journal once again, and attempt to complete this, our piece of work. As I share events, always keep the *illness* in mind, not my special person, David Kimball. He and I have read most of these chapters together during some of his lucid times and his response has always been the same: "If it can help someone else, write it down. That may be part of God's purpose in allowing me to have to cope with it."

I cannot quite imagine the portion of each and every day that is allotted to turmoil control. The necessity for spontaneous plans to handle issues while they are still manageable is always before me. Hot spots become a way of life from waking 'til bedtime, blessed bedtime! Each day centers around avoidance mode. It is a major challenge to find enough things to fill the hours during which Dave can get into trouble.

I dream up ways that get Dave away from the consistently frustrating and sterile atmosphere his home and his life present to him, so far as any productive activity is concerned. He often wanders from room to room, restless and bored, wondering how to endure the hours from now 'til bedtime. I hear his deep sighs. They seem more like suppressed moans. My immediate concern is how to be supportive.

The car helps, and compared to a year ago we are spending more and more time there. We go to the ocean; we do one errand, saving another as an excuse for tomorrow; we go for a ride in the country. We go for coffee.

That mention of coffee is becoming a major prop for a difficult morning as it seems to present a bright new focus. "Let's go for coffee," I suggest. "Good idea," is always his eager response, and even his voice changes quality. Best of all, if he is struggling with something that he feels is especially difficult, he forgets it immediately.

Our daughters abet the solution by keeping cash in the "MAD MONEY" jar, bless their hearts! They also tuck gift certificates into that jar for visits to nearby eating spots. They can't imagine how those little pieces of paper help us get through another long day. I am sure I am connecting with some of my fellow caregivers. Perhaps you could use the above idea as a gift suggestion among your family.

If I leave enough slack time for Dave to become creative, he will usually try to find something that needs fixing, which predictably ends up in some sort of chaos. I try to watch, too often unsuccessfully, anything that can be disassembled. Our family den is now without one of its table lamps. It sits on the work bench sans shade, bulb, socket or wire, only a stem and base, looking quite lonely and useless. Someday I'll reassemble it -- if I can. Dave must have decided one day that it needed fixing. Beside it lies his sander, now in several parts, another victim of fixing.

One of our nice antique Seth Thomas oak schoolroom clocks fell into the same fateful category. I was alerted by the sound of hammering. Upon investigating I found Dave replacing the face of the clock (why had he taken it off?) by hammering nails into it, while the tiny screws he had removed lay in plain sight where he had placed them moments before. I cringed in dismay and rescued the clock.

If he disappears from the room for long I may find him in the bathroom, searching through the cabinets. For what? He usually has no idea. It is just something to do. Of necessity I have removed all liquid items from the bathroom vanity. A variety of bottles such as contact lens solution, mineral oil, rubbing alcohol, began appearing on Dave's night stand. He "had no idea how they got there."

I long ago hid all medications. He has not yet found my hiding place. If he finds my caches I will have to put things elsewhere, or buy a lock for a cabinet. I have not considered locks so far. I want to avoid his feeling shut out of something else in his life.

Dave seldom forgets to shave, a leftover from his impeccable grooming days. But he occasionally forgets where he shaves, or where he keeps his razor. This sends him on an endless search through cabinets, drawers, and shelves, unless I intervene and remind him where to look. Sometimes I just let him search. It takes up some of his time and gives him something to do. So sad for my Valedictorian husband.

Eventually, after he began cutting himself with his safety razor, we replaced it with an electric model, which he promptly took apart. Predictable, but I forgot to pay attention. Our good neighbor, George, was able to reassemble it.

Dave then tried using his stick deodorant as a shaving cream. Cleaning the razor from all that "goo" was another challenge. I forthwith put the deodorant away after each use, along with the rest of the hidden items, and saw to it that I was the one who cleaned the razor each day. This, of course, meant one more thing to watch so as to know when he was finished, and before the disassembling process had a chance to start. The razor was then added to my sizable cache of hidden items.

Another part of Dave's impeccable grooming was his nicely polished shoes. They were always one of his trademarks. Now he has no concept of the amount of polish he is using, and he forgets the buffing. The rug in front of his chair, plus smaller areas in other rooms are often smeared with polish. Result? Carpet cleaner and hide the shoe polish. One big problem -- I now have so much hidden that I can't remember my hiding places. But one thing is certain. If Dave ever looks under my bed he will think Christmas is coming!

Just the putting out of the trash has to be supervised. It very often goes out on the wrong day, and must be retrieved. Each container has to be looked over to be sure nothing of value is on its way to the dump. Dave feels degraded. "What are you doing?", he will ask. "Making sure there is nothing here that shouldn't be thrown away," I reply. "Honestly, anyone would think I didn't have a brain," Dave will often respond. A cloud drops over my heart. I say something like, "We all make mistakes, Dear." Does that compensate for his hurt feelings? I don't know.

Alzheimer's also accompanies us to restaurants. Menus for Dave are a maze. Selecting from them and remembering that selection until the waitress returns is impossible for him to manage alone. Once he has selected, we take the menu and keep it out of sight. Otherwise, he will go over and over it, not remembering that he has made a choice. When the waitress comes we order for him, and we usually explain why. Doing so seems more kind than allowing him to struggle and become embarrassed over his inadequacy.

Increasingly he no longer remembers that he has eaten, so after enjoying a hearty meal he thinks he is still hungry and would raid the refrigerator if we did not remind him. He gives in reluctantly. "Are you sure?", he asks, skeptically.

Knowing where his clothes belong is a lost art. He usually forgets where to hang his coat when he comes in from outdoors, and shows great displeasure if I remind him. It constitutes just another invasion into his manhood and independence. But picture the search when he wants one certain coat which could be in any one of three closets. He does the same thing with his sweaters.

When he is too warm he may leave on either coat or sweater and open a window. We joke that his temperature tolerance has a variance now of about 3 degrees. At 71° we need the furnace turned up (I sometimes find the thermostat on 90°); at 74° we need the air conditioner on! That subject is now becoming more problem than joke. I must check the thermostat constantly. Unfortunately it is on the way to his room and he seems to feel the need to do something to it each time he passes.

He is beginning to lose track of family members, some of whom are no longer living, such as his brother Bob, who has been in Heaven for several years. When we go to Karen's home he confuses it with one belonging to a departed cousin Eleanor, and can no longer figure out why the name plate, K. S. Kimball is on Eleanor's door. Yet, he usually knows Karen while we are there, but forgets her, and where we have been, as soon as we leave. One night recently he said on the way home, "It sure is nice to have Eleanor near by. I wonder what made her move way out here." He thought we were still living in Illinois. We hadn't lived there for forty years.

One night we went to Michelle's so I could help her with a project which happened to be upstairs. We had decided on diversion for Dave which would occupy him 'til we were finished. The seat of one of Michelle's dining room chairs still needed its old upholstery replaced. This was an easy job. Dave just had to take out four good-sized screws, and remove the upholsterers tacks from the bottom of the seat. We set him up in the kitchen and went upstairs to do our thing.

A short time later I decided I should check on his progress. As I came into the kitchen I noted a pile of screws on the table. A lot more than just four! I asked, "Where did all the screws come from?" "From the other chairs," replied Dave. Sure enough, he had taken the other chairs apart.

Unfortunately, screw holes in each chair matched only the seat that belonged with it. Michelle and I exchanged glances. We got Dave back on his project, and she and I started matching up screw holes. Dave didn't have a clue. Eventually we succeeded, Dave finished with the tacks, the new piece of upholstery went on, and we placed the chairs back in the dining room. Project accomplished, though by a somewhat later hour than we had planned. Dave still without a clue.

As we said goodnight at the door Michelle thanked Dave for all his help. Dave smiled graciously with much gratitude for her thanks and replied, "You're welcome, Honey. I'm glad to help any time I can."

But my greatest burden, day after endless day, concerns Dave's most frustrating adjustment concerning the garage. Once his playhouse, it now has to be kept locked. This engendered a huge conflict. I would awake every morning knowing it would be another day of bitterness and fury, knowing he would head out the door by 8:15 or so; knowing he would be back in a few minutes for the garage key; and knowing the strife my response was going to ignite. How I dreaded getting up in the morning.

The locking became necessary due to Dave's inability to reason that there were things out there that mustn't be taken apart, stored up on the rafters out of my reach, discarded, or that didn't require rewiring. Twice he attempted to rewire the garage itself, and in so doing left it without lights, and with hot wires exposed. In his altered state of reasoning he could not understand why that mattered. I was meddling with his manhood again. It was indeed a challenge to attempt to explain this affront so that although he could no longer understand it, he would accept it.

That inevitable question, "Where is the garage key?", asked multiple times a day, sometimes six days a week, and for weeks on end, spawned many a storm. Upon being refused, he would leave the house in a rage, and in a very few minutes would have forgotten that he had just been through that. Back in the house for a repeat of the same performance, over and over again.

Often his next step was to gather up all the stray keys in the house and try every single one, hoping to outwit me and find a fit. The failure only increased his rage.

There were times when I could have imagined that the garage door might be demolished in order for him to gain entrance into *his domain*. There were also times when I expected he would become violent toward me. He would sidle up to me threateningly and with a fiery glare in his eye, demand that key. Awful Alzheimer's.

Dr. Fiori once said to me, "I am going to ask you a straight question and I want a straight answer. When David becomes so angry has he ever smacked you?" I was able to answer "no" truthfully, though I did admit to having backed up a step on one occasion. "If he ever does," Dr. Fiori said, "we're dealing with a whole new ball game."

After many months the issue subsided, mainly because Dr. Fiori prescribed medication to calm down the anger when in desperation I finally cried for help. As soon as I detected undue stress I offered medication, and if it was refused I slipped it into a cup of coffee which was seldom refused. If it was, I placed the cup nearby with a silent prayer, and thankfully he usually drank it as soon as I was out of sight. Medication kept that part of our journey from becoming totally unmanageable.

How I dislike my role. It can foster a terrible load of the guilties. But the result of the medication was rewarding for us both: a change of pace for me; a good nap for Dave; after which the subject was forgotten -- for a while.

Now, Dave exhibits a restrained and somewhat bewildered resignation over the subject, but seems content to let it be that way. Most of the time I don't get those butterflies in my tummy upon hearing the back door open, as I did when I knew I was going to hear that inevitable question again, and handle that anger again, over and over for yet another long day. For this I can only be terribly grateful.

A strange sequel to this story is that in the midst of one of Dave's blackest and most unreachable moods, Michelle can walk in and the mood immediately disappears. My old Dave is suddenly present, gracious, kind, and cooperative. I shake my head as I am suddenly confronted with feelings of -- what? Inadequacy?

Many other miscellania come to mind but these will suffice to indicate the unreal, even extreme, events which stealthily creep in and make up the world in which we of the Alzheimer's community, *in fact,* do live, move, and have our being.

Chapter 25

ALONE

I have just returned from a week at the place of my roots, that place of loons and wild blueberries among other things, by lovely Lake Pennamaquan, where my brother and I spent those first five years of our lives, and which comes closer to being home to us than any other place on earth. I am now 78. My roots are still there.

As I anticipated the week with my husband I wondered to myself just what this time at "Camp," would produce in my heart and mind. The mere passage of several years since we were last there by ourselves, the addition of Dave's illness which produces in him an uneasiness when away from things familiar, my difficulty in handling the rougher landscape there, coping with things like less-than-easy bathroom facilities -- these and other items did not escape my contemplation as we departed on our nine-hour drive to this lovely isolated place deep in Washington County, Maine, town of Charlotte.

We arrived at 7 PM, just in time to avoid the onslaught of mosquitoes which appear at dusk. Three loons were fishing for their supper in the little cove by our beach. They obviously noted our arrival but seemed not to be perturbed by our presence.

We unpacked the car, readied our beds with our sleeping bags and retired early. In the old days our grandparents often let darkness dictate bed time. Consequently rising time was early -- a lovely time of day.

Birds were welcoming the sunrise with zestful enthusiasm as we awoke the next morning, and our friends the loons were already cruising, this time for their breakfast. Their babies, upon wearying with the process, occasionally opted for a restful piggyback ride on the back of a parent. One of my favorite sights.

The arrival of each new day restarted the constant process of getting, and keeping, Dave oriented to this new place. All personal daily functions were being carried out in a new location, and all accessories were, of course, in new places, all of which was beyond his memory from day to day. Finding his way to the bathroom at night for his several visits required the attention of both of us.

I had envisioned lengthy periods of reading on the veranda, but Dave's attention to books is becoming sketchy and brief. That left us with the problem of "what to do." TV reception is poor, Dave deplores jig-saw puzzles, and can no longer understand games.

So we spent much of our time away from camp enjoying happy times with old friends, satiating ourselves with all kinds of wonderful sea food, and on a few brief occasions we did manage to languish in the pristine beauty all around us from the vantage point of the screened veranda, especially when we had our morning coffee.

But I made some discoveries about myself that week. It was a time for shedding tears. Shed privately at night when Dave was asleep. They were tears of sadness, due to a sense of loss of what had been, of what had changed, and of what could not be reproduced; tears because, even with a telephone, I suddenly felt alone for the first time ever, down there in the woods, a bright moon shining on a lovely lake where the silhouettes of trees and hilltops were starkly familiar; tears because the man who lay sleeping so close by could no longer be my head and my protector; could not even undertake the normal functions of staying clean or of remembering the new place to go to the bathroom.

Even the loons seemed to confirm my confused emotions by alternately laughing and crying during several of those nights. They too sounded as if they were making emotional decisions, down there at the foot of the lake, the jubilant yeas on the one hand, the mournful nays on the other. Those of you who have had the privilege of hearing those sounds know what I mean.

But my tears produced some much-needed reality thinking, starting with the realization that my desire for remembering this cherished place could be pretty much satisfied by my own vivid memories. And to assist my memories is a lovely picture of the things that seem important to remember, a picture painted recently by my brother Harry, a very fine artist. From his own memory of those early days and with the help of some very old snapshots, his picture includes the cottage, always called "Camp," Grampa's woodpile, his flag pole, our swing hanging between two white birches, Nana's patch of pond lillies, Rocky Point, a sail boat, MacGregor's boat pier, and the railroad track, among other things. The picture hangs in our "Camp" room at home, a room where we enjoy the warmth of the old stove that once served as the single heat source at this spot where we once lived.

I further realized that I did not need to be here in body, trying to pretend that things were the same, and that I could cope in the way I always had. Hips and knees don't meet the challenge as they once did, of hillsides, rough terrain, and steps without railings. Porta-potties need emptying, spring water does not last forever if the faucet is left running, etc., etc. And the need for one person to do the thinking for two and keep an Alzheimer's patient occupied is much less an encumbrance in more simple and familiar surroundings.

I was suddenly gripped with the reality that my support people were 400 miles away. I felt a surge of need to have them closer. That could only be accomplished by readying the car with all our belongings, closing Camp by myself, and then facing that 400 mile return trip back to where they were. Dave is no longer able to help with even the simplest functions, so it all felt like another very long day to me.

Suddenly the word aloneness took on a whole new meaning to me. I have never minded being alone. In fact, in the light of our people-oriented existence in the pastorate for 30 years I rather enjoy just my own company occasionally. But being alone became a stark reality during those seven days at the lake.

Aloneness took on two faces, one face being the bodily, physical part, and the other the intellectual and emotional. The role of the caregiver makes bodily and physical aloneness virtually non-existent, yet, personally, you are still always alone. It is a strange paradox, and one which I am sure hundreds of caregivers would readily confirm. My only real aloneness during each long day is accomplished during Dave's one hour nap in the afternoon, and following his bedtime at 9 P.M. Even then the responsibilities are always present. You are alone, yet you aren't.

But the other aloneness, the intellectual and emotional, settled in like a dead weight up there in the lovely Maine woods. Any attempt at conversation, with routine predictability, went nowhere except into bewilderment and confusion for Dave, and frustration for me. It served only to emphasize how shrunken our capacity for communication had become, and it underscored the stark reality of that impersonal world in which caregivers must increasingly learn to exist. I had wanted to make these days a continuation of what I had always experienced there at Camp. It did not work.

Personal survival depends upon a caregiver facing the necessary changes due to circumstances, in my opinion. As I have said before, nothing is static in lives affected by this illness, and facing changes suddenly included the role that Camp had played in my life since birth. Finally I realized I must allow Camp to exist in memory alone, except for an occasional visit with other family members who could be there to help.

A monumental decision gradually formed in my mind in the middle of the night, monumental because of what this location has always meant to me. With that decision I found myself transferring the place of my roots into its own quiet resting place. I resolved never to do this again -- come here, just the two of us, and try to manage in my aloneness.

That resolve, though accomplished in the midst of an intense emotional struggle, was liberating beyond words. There were no more tears. The sadness dissipated. There emerged a calmness of spirit which seemed not quite real but which has continued to comfort me in its quiet way through the weeks following our return home. I repeatedly contemplate my decision. I look up at my picture. I reminisce with my brother about that nostalgic place, and my heart is at rest.

I leave Camp as a part of family history and I sense no need for further reflection. The decision must simply be accepted as the result of another inroad by the ever-dominant presence of Alzheimer's. How it does change lives.

Gwen Bibber Kimball

Chapter 26

CALLING A SPADE A SPADE

With no regrets, actually with great relief on my part, we left the place of my roots about ten o'clock on a bright sunny morning. I was happy to be heading home. The car was loaded, everything was turned off and closed up, and Dave had spent his considerable time in the bathroom. He had emerged with comments of great success. I was glad. That event was out of the way.

Once upon a time I would have considered this subject to be one of the most private areas of ones life, not one to be introduced in a chapter of a book. I still consider it so, but this is the illness, Alzheimer's, we are talking about, not the person, and Alzheimer's invades all privacy. Unfortunately, preoccupation with this subject is common with this illness. In honesty and fairness it must be introduced, or the picture of care is not complete.

It is not unusual for the victim to spend much time in the bathroom, forgetting that "he has been there, done that."

Such was the case with Dave. He had turned the bathroom into a Library. His multiple visits, along with one of his books, was becoming a training ground for constantly having to be there. Each nonproductive visit was deemed to be the "need for some prunes." He totally lost sight of his once-normal habit of one visit a day.

Recently I heard of a theory which explained the function of a small portion of the brain which is one's internal clock. In Lab animals, when that portion was removed, the time clock was totally inoperable. In humans, if that portion was surgically removed it affected the sense of timing of when to eat, when to be active, when to sleep. It also regulated the sense of needing to go to the bathroom. Any experience in caregiving attests to these problems.

If Alzheimer's, which leaves its victims with no *memory* of having gone to the bathroom, also affects the portion of the brain which indicates ones *need* to go, as well as the appropriate *time* to go, then the victim is in triple jeopardy. Perhaps this explains why Dave is so often found in the reading room, again, at 2 AM or so.

This had been a developing problem for months. It indeed had become a fetish. Reasoning was useless. It only created resentment and temper. In a wild moment I had even considered locking the bathroom door in the hope that the lack of availability might discourage the practice. Common sense told me that was an extreme measure and would only provoke more fury on Dave's part. I find that this illness has the propensity for causing caregivers to entertain irresponsible thoughts.

The week at Camp was no exception to what had become commonplace at home: off to the little room with the book for ten or fifteen minutes. Shortly, if we were in town, it was *find a bathroom*, day after day. I made many side trips and we stopped often for another cup of coffee, simply because there was a bathroom available.

Yet, I knew that diversion was a factor. If his attention was taken from the subject he would forget it, sometimes for hours.

Such was my hope for our trip home, and I was glad for Dave's earlier bathroom visit at Camp. The first two hours would take us along the heavily wooded, sparsely settled Rt. 9, a route nicknamed "The Airline." It had provided pilots with a general easterly route from Bangor during those days when navigational aids were few. It was once a winding, rutty, gravel road, passable for the earliest cars only during dry months. It is now a good road for most of its ninety miles, though there are few stops on that long stretch from Camp.

As we made our way west and stopped for lunch at noon, the inevitable happened. Dave headed for the men's room before we were even seated. In our early days Dave never would have left me standing. He would have seated me first. After some length of time, during which I finally found a chair, he emerged exclaiming triumphantly about his successful visit. I thought to myself, "That's twice."

Later on, about 2:30 in the afternoon, we stopped on the Maine Turnpike for an ice cream cone. Dave predictably headed for the men's room again, leaving me standing in the foyer -- again. I thought to myself, "That's three times."

Again I waited, and I waited. Again I found a chair and waited some more. I finally went to the men's room door, opened it a tiny crack and called his name. He answered, sounding a bit stressed. Finally he came out looking less than triumphant.

We purchased our cones, returned to the car, and once again got on the road. As we did so Dave said, "I don't know what's wrong, but I think I need some prunes."

Reality came crashing in on me. It was a bare, gut-level reality. It was a reality I had been desperately trying to ignore for months. I felt angry. I felt victimized. I felt helpless.

I began to cry. I literally shouted! "What a cockamamie comment; how stupid; how ridiculous; that's got to be the dumbest thing you ever said in your whole life," etc., etc. The words came in torrents, and I spouted on and cried for fifteen minutes, I suppose. I really don't know how long it all lasted.

By the time I was spent I was absolutely silent for an hour. I just doggedly drove. As I drove I did a lot of thinking about this reality that had come crashing in on me. Why had I reacted the way I did? What was this that had clobbered me so fiercely?

The reality was that *this is the way things are. I cannot ignore this plain fact any longer, much as I would like to. This is Alzheimer's. This behavior and these dumb remarks are not Dave Kimball and he is not my foe. I have been finding it impossible to give in to this fact, but I must. Could he, who has been so bright, become so unintelligent? Yes, he could, and he has, and I must accept it. This is the best he can do!*

That was my crushing reality, and crushing it was. I suppose sooner or later that dreaded reality had to really dawn on me in a more final way than at any time before. I was not prepared for it to be so devastating.

Finally I took his hand and I sobbed out an apology for my behavior. I so needed him to say, "I forgive you, Dear. I know you didn't mean all that."

Dave, by now, didn't even know what I was referring to, and had forgotten my tirade. His response? "I want to make things as easy for you as possible," a statement he had made, word for word on many occasions, and pertaining to many subjects. It was a rote reply, addressing nothing in particular.

My apology felt ignored and discarded, though I knew that had not been Dave's intent. With my apology, however, came relief for me from the guilt of my inordinate fury and frustration. And with that crushing reality my suit of armor called denial had been shattered. I felt released. I would now be better able to handle other irrational realities as they continually inserted themselves into our lives.

In my opinion, born of a hard lesson learned, all caregivers must accept and face, sooner or later, the fact that denial only prolongs the agony and increases the stress.

I held Dave's hand for a lot of miles that day, as we continued our long trip home.

A postscript: I called Dr. Fiori and recounted my episode. He said, "Good. You will need a safety-valve along the way, on occasion. Don't be too hard on yourself if that happens."

I thanked him for his support and understanding, but of course I was not pleased with myself, nor am I planning other temper tantrums in my future. Now that my wall of denial, which I had used as a protection against the pain of stark realities, has been breached, I believe I shall be better able to recognize stark realities and face them headon. I had not realized how often I was using denial to protect myself, until this event.

It was a true wake-up call.

Gwen Bibber Kimball

Chapter 27

LOST GLASSES

This saga came about because the bow came off my reading glasses, presenting me with the need for the right size tiny little screw, or a new pair of glasses. I opted for a new pair after spending entirely too much time trying to find a screw that would fit that tiny hole. Dropping screw after screw on the table, picking them up with my stiff fingers and starting over with others, which also did not fit, sent me on my way to a simpler solution.

Together with Dave at about 12:30 one midday I decided to take a brief jaunt to a store named Building 19, a place known for its bargains.

There were bargains, but something happened to the brief jaunt part. After scanning the racks and finding nothing for me, we went on to a local CVS drug store. On our way to the reading glass rack Dave spied the sunglasses. He stopped there. I assumed no harm could come from his being such a short distance away from me for a few moments so I went on to the reading glasses.

After some careful searching I gave up and went back to where Dave was, only to find him looking upset. Upon my questioning he responded that he had been looking at sunglasses and now he couldn't find his own regular glasses. They were bifocals, new only two months ago, and it would appear that they were hopelessly lost somewhere among 100 or so pairs on those two racks in front of us.

The following two hours went something like this: (please keep in mind that Dave now wore two hearing aids).

"Did you walk away from here and lay them down on another shelf somewhere?"

Dave: "What?"

Repeat.

Dave: "No, I stayed right here." I could only hope he remembered correctly. No guarantees of that, however.

We started a search, hoping that he had tucked his glasses into an empty space once occupied by a pair that had been sold. Through both racks. No glasses.

I asked, "Do you have them in a pocket?"

Dave: "'What?"

Repeat.

He said, "No." Just in case he had missed something in a pocket, I searched. No glasses.

I went to the cashier. "Did anyone turn in a pair of glasses? My husband seems to have lost his around the sunglass racks."

The cashier said no, nothing had been turned in, so I left our name and telephone number and asked her to call if they turned up.

I asked Dave if he was sure he had been wearing them. "Yes, he was sure." "No, he wasn't sure."

I then explained that perhaps we should go home and search for them there. After the necessary explaining and repeating he understood, and we started home.

On the way I said, "Perhaps they got left at Building 19."

Dave said, "What?"

I repeated.

Dave: "Where?"

"Building 19."

Dave: "We didn't go there."

"Yes, we did. We looked there first."

Dave: "What?"

"We looked there first."

Dave: "I have no memory of that."

"Well, we did. Take my word for it."

Dave: "Maybe. I don't remember that. Why would we go there?"

"To look for some reading glasses for me."

Dave: "What?"

"To look for some reading glasses for me."

Dave: "Well, I have no memory of it."

"Well, let's just say that I do. But we'll look at home first."

Dave: "What?"

I responded with a wave of my hand and a "Never mind."

Dave: "Well, why are you being that way?"

I made no response.

We arrived home and searched the house. No glasses. I asked, "Did you happen to look downstairs?"

Dave: "What for?"

"Your glasses." I looked downstairs. No glasses. So I said, "Let's go back to Building 19."

Dave: "Why?"

"To find your glasses."

Dave: "If you say so. Just wait 'til I go get my glasses."

"They're lost. That's why we're going to Building 19!"

Dave: "O. K., but why don't we just get an appointment and get a new pair?"

"Because they're only two months old and they cost money."

Dave: "That's what I mean." (?)

By now I was becoming mildly frantic. I had a sudden impulse to do something clever with a handful of hair, but not having been overly endowed in that department I decided against it. Better to just get in the car and go on back to Building 19.

The clerk there was very helpful, but there were no glasses. So I decided to go back to CVS without any announcements. Easier that way. I also decided that I would go in by myself and bypass the question and answer periods.

Upon arriving at the store I said, "You wait here and I'll be back shortly."

Dave: "What?"

Repeat.

Dave: "Why?"

"It will be easier this way." I turned off the motor, took the keys, put my purse in the trunk and went into CVS. The cashier had had no glasses turned in.

I went over and over those racks, believing those glasses HAD to be there somewhere. Maybe inside a clip-on envelope. No. Maybe I missed them. Over and over. No. Maybe they are inside a clip-on envelope with clip-ons on them. No. Maybe they are on a rack with a pair of clip-ons on them, making them look like regular sunglasses. EUREKA!!

I went to the cashier, brandishing my find, thanked her, and returned to the car, and triumphantly presented the glasses.

Dave: "What's this?"

"Your glasses."

Dave: "Where were they?"

"On the rack with sunglasses attached to them."

Dave: "What?"

Repeat.

Dave: "So it was a very normal mistake."

"Sure. It's O.K. You don't need to feel defensive."

Dave: "I'm not feeling defensive. I'm just glad you found your glasses."

By now it was nearing three o'clock. I was worn to the place of not knowing whether to laugh at this ridiculous episode, or to cry from sheer frustration. Besides, my hip hurt! And I still had no reading glasses.

I called Karen to recount, and give vent to, the past two and one-half hours of my life. She asked, "Mom, are you laughing or crying?" I wasn't too sure. I only knew that this was just another day in the life of the caregiver and her very dear, and very deaf, Alzheimer's-victim husband.

Gwen Bibber Kimball

Chapter 28

WIDOWHOOD

I started the year 2000 feeling my way into a sort of "widowhood," a path I had been becoming acquainted with for several years. Since the advent of Dave's Alzheimer's, life had very gradually produced a sense of solitary-ness for each of us. For Dave it was a decline into a distant world. For me it was a gradual cessation of being a wife, a companion, a part of a team. There were still two of us, but the team seldom functioned as such. I pondered the somewhat vague feelings of widowhood many times as I gradually became aware of them.

But the days presented no crises which would make those feelings sharp and poignant until January 2nd when Dave was hospitalized with pneumonia. He had fallen five times the night before, all the while his temperature rising, so I knew he was in trouble. He was transported by ambulance from his bedroom floor where he had lain on an egg-crate pad, covered with a comforter, asleep since his last fall. Michelle, Karen and I could no longer help him up.

The girls stayed by me all day in the Emergency Room until we finally returned to our homes in the early evening. Karen stayed with me. As I walked in and closed the door behind me and felt the feelings of occupying our home all by myself without Dave, the reality was stark. I felt like a widow. Not a grieving widow. Just an emotionless widow.

There comes a time when weariness and relief go hand in hand. So, no, I did not grieve when I walked in. I felt only a vast relief; relief at being alone; relief that I was "off-duty" for a few days; relief that I could sit down and get up when I wanted to; relief that I could go to bed when I wanted to; relief that I could read or type when I wanted to. This has nothing to do with love; it has a lot to do with survival. It has nothing to do with the person who has been my life and my companion for 58+ years; it has everything to do with Alzheimer's.

In tears, I breathed a huge sigh and said to Karen, "Can you imagine! A few days with no responsibilities." I could turn off my internal alarm system. I could leave my toilet articles, comb and mirror in plain sight on the vanity and not have to hide them under my bed. I could come and go without making sure that Dave was dressed appropriately, and that he had recently been to the bathroom, etc. I would not have to keep a watchful eye on activities from morn 'til night, with the possibility of unpleasant confrontations which so easily, and all too often, ensue. Evenings would be mine, without the two-hour stress of trying to keep Dave from retiring to his bed at seven o'clock instead of nine (with the consequence of his being up in the morning at four instead of six). I would not have to be up several times in the night and be on deck so early. I could also go to bed and go to sleep without one ear open. Widowhood from Alzheimer's. How completely that illness invades lives.

Being alone also felt like being on vacation. The best word to describe it was the word free. Free from my existence alongside that huge gulf which is so effectively separating me from my introverted stranger. Suddenly I felt as if I had escaped it all; was beyond it all; was away from it all. Widowhood. I must confess to an enormous sense of reprieve. I felt no guilt.

In consideration of the quality of Dave's life, and the need for me to somehow handle his increasing descent into the unawareness of who he is, and what he is about, I found myself praying in quiet desperation, "Lord, if it be your will, during this illness please take Dave out of his morass and lift him to Heaven." Our family joined me in that prayer, and we felt free to ask close friends to do the same.

My prayers were not accompanied by the deep sorrow which would be present with those who have no hope. If I believe what I say I believe, then Heaven is an especially prepared place for God's children. He tells us that so clearly in I Corinthians 2:9 when He says that "no mere man has ever seen, heard, or even imagined what wonderful things God has ready for those who love the Lord" (LB). When that day comes that Dave enters into the Presence of Jesus I expect to find my sorrow outweighed by sheer joy at his liberation from feeling brainless, useless, and helpless.

However, as we prayed for God's will, back at the hospital Dave was in fact recovering. The days progressed from the predicted three, to seven. During those days it was necessary to have a sitter with him constantly, day and night. He was confused, uncooperative, angry and combative. It was a constant challenge to keep him in bed and keep his various tubes in place.

At the end of the seven days he had recovered from the pneumonia and was in a calmer state, due to medication. However, it appeared that he had developed a urinary incontinence. He was transferred to a short-term Rehabilitation Center and I was being encouraged to place him in long-term care. The professionals felt I had done my tour of duty and that it was time to consider other arrangements, mainly for me as a caregiver.

That advice placed upon me the need to make some decisions. Does Dave come home again? Can he be medicated so that he will sleep at night, permitting me to sleep also? Is he in fact incontinent? Will he resort to his former displeasure and borderline anger when he is crossed, as has been the growing pattern for some time? Will he need such things as bed-rails? Can I go back to all the problems inherent with his living at home? I thought about the liberation I had felt. I reminded myself again that I am 78+ years old.

Dave's new medication continued to keep him remarkably calm, and his incontinence proved to be a matter of confusion as to where the bathroom was, in new surroundings. But at night he slept fitfully and roamed the corridors a great deal. Many evenings when I left him he cried and pleaded to come home with me "where it was safe." I, of course, left by myself and cried all the way home.

In order to be prepared for all possibilities, the next step seemed to be a matter of at least investigating various nursing homes, specifically those dealing with Dave's illness. I set about becoming aware of what was out there. The one I would have preferred was not a locked home, and was surrounded by water. Lovely, but for Dave, dangerous. I asked questions about several others from knowledgeable people, and Karen and I finally arranged a visit for the following day to a highly recommended home that dealt with only Alzheimer's patients.

The evening before that visit was a highly traumatic one for me. I was contemplating the finality of Dave's never being in our home another night after 58+ years. I considered the choice of grieving my way through the night alone, or of going home with Karen. She has a guest room she calls "Mom's room." My judgment told me that being alone would be nonproductive, even though part of me wanted to just sit and grieve. Reluctantly I decided to go with Karen and occupy my room there. I'm sure it was the better decision, even though she did beat me at multiple games of Rummikub.

As we toured the nursing home the next day we found a clean, cheerful facility, beautifully decorated, well staffed, with obviously well-cared-for patients. But we found no patient with the amount of awareness that Dave still has. He is, as yet, very aware of his need for privacy. He still needs time to be alone with his books and videos, his pictures and his treasures. He is not a Bingo person, nor is he interested, in the least, in occupational therapy. He would have been frantic!

I am not a person who has cried her way through life, but I cried much of the way through the tour. I cried all the way home. I sat in my chair and cried. Karen comforted me as best she could but I was beside myself. My friend Donna, who had guided us through the facility had said, "God will show you what to do." He did. An immediate and overwhelming conviction was pressing down upon me. There was no way I would sleep in peace another night of my life knowing that Dave, with his amount of awareness, was deposited into one of those three-beds-to-a-room settings, no matter how nice the facility, to spend the remainder of his life. I vowed that when that event comes, it will be only when he no longer knows who he is and what he is about, as long as I remain able.

As simply as that my mind was made up. And out of the blue, in walked two dear friends who always seem to produce fun and light-heartedness. In my book "You say WHAT, Lord?", I speak often of the *special angels* God sent into our lives at just the right moment. These two were my special angels for that night in my life. They could not have been sent at a better time. How up-close and personal our Father is!

We visited and laughed a while, as is always the case with Barbara and Eddie. I patched up my red eyes, and they took us out to eat. My heart was at rest and I knew that, for now, I had no more questions about nursing homes. Get Dave on adequate sleeping medication and he would come home, period. The relief that had accompanied my being free of caregiving was overtaken by the desire for Dave's future to be as quality as possible for as long as we could manage, together. Feelings of widowhood receded into the background, due partly, I am sure, to my 17 days of change and rest.

At the Rehabilitation Center I pressed for more attention to Dave's sleeping needs. Five nights later, after he had slept all night on a combination of Haldol and Trazadone with only one interruption, we cheered. He came home that day, January 18th.

I took up my mantle again. Within a few hours he had no memory of ever having been away.

Michelle and Karen were unwavering in their presence and support the entire time. I could not have handled it without them. That first week at the Rehabilitation Center was the worst week of my life. I knew the subject of long-term care would be difficult, but I had no idea how emotional it would become.

Our dear approachable Dr. Fiori is available to make medication changes as necessary. He assures me that, "I am here and have no plans to go away." I am to call him in a heart-beat. What security and comfort!

The entire experience provided for me a time to learn and reassess. It was during that time that God suggested I needed to rearrange my priorities. Many issues must become non-issues. I am working on that.

My personal things are back in hiding, and for some reason I don't seem to mind much. I will do less protesting when Dave rummages in the drawers.

And finally I found myself face to face with the catalyst for settling the garden issue. After experiencing the possibility of placing Dave in a nursing home, those gardens suddenly became entirely unimportant. They would be fixable later on. I would say nothing, ever again, when he tramps.

I did whimper a bit to myself the first time he strode purposefully through the shrubs which were brittle with the below-freezing temperatures, but I ignored it. And though I must admit to subtle twinges of feeling most noble and virtuous, sudden recall of "nursing home" reminded me of my goal. Why do we always have to have such trouble with our humanness?

And so we go on, comfortably for now. For how long? One doesn't ask questions like that when dealing with Alzheimer's. We shall see. For the present, Dave is home once again. This time he is quiet, controlled and manageable with his new medications. They have changed our lives.

And I am back to tucking him in at night and saying, "Good night, Dear, see you in the morning."

Chapter 29

OUR LAST THREE MONTHS

Dave's hospitalization in January became a blessing to both of us because of the medication changes. He continues to be calm and pleasant, sort of a restoration of my old Dave, and he continues to sleep at night. This is more than I could have hoped for at this stage of his illness.

His daily care is presenting new duties, however, as the days pass. He is slowly becoming unable to dress himself. His arms can't seem to find his shirt and sweater sleeves, and I must help him get his socks on, and tie his shoes. Buttons and button holes usually don't come out even. I remember seeing an elderly, very dignified doctor on the street one day with his jacket askew because he had not noticed the problem with the buttons. I felt so sorry about that. Now it is my honor-student husband who no longer notices. I have come to a solution for his almost continuously soiled underwear. I found a very thin pad of a good size, with an adhesive strip to keep it in place inside his shorts. I was washing and bleaching his shorts constantly, sometimes as many as twelve or fourteen a week.

With the pads I have only to remove the pad, make sure he is clean, and reinsert a fresh pad. He wears them day and night with no complaints. I would recommend them heartily for anyone with the slightest problem of fecal incontinence.

I also found a foam cleanser in a spray can, a pleasant aroma, and not expensive. Using it on bathroom tissue, in place of soap and water and a face cloth, is infinitely easier and more effective, usually requiring only one application of the foam, and drying with fresh tissue. This has made a major change in what was a tedious project -- keeping Dave clean and fresh.

His personal price for all this, however, is the invasion of his bathroom privacy which must be painful for him. He stands mute while I care for him. I try to restore a bit of his ego when I am finished by exclaiming, "Ooh, you smell so good -- like my Dave." He makes no response but, again, I can only hope it helps his feelings.

Dave's unsteadiness in the shower, and his inability to turn the shower head in the right direction caused us to make some changes and additions. We had grab bars installed, and finally added a seat. He feels more secure with the seat, though he objected to having to make another change in routine.

I never seem able to find just the right temperature for the water. He either shouts, in fear that it is too hot, or shivers and says it is freezing, although it feels right to me. But after a few trials we do quite well, and he agrees that he feels safer.

He no longer remembers that after a shower you dry off with a towel, so I gladly give him a good rubdown and care for his feet. I had felt gratified that the nurses commented on how immaculate he was the day he was admitted to the hospital.

After this new shower routine was adopted, I, of course, reaped the benefit of no longer having to mop up water from all over the bathroom. Dave had lost all sense of direction with the shower head and the results were widespread!

He who was always so fussy about being clean-shaven is now slowly forgetting about shaving at all, and is losing any awareness of what to shave. One cheek often is red from the constant rubbing in one spot, while the other portions of his face go totally unnoticed. He exhibits an amazing amount of grace and patience while I finish this chore for him in a manner totally unlike anything he is accustomed to, I'm sure. I try to take the curse off by doing a cheek to cheek with a satisfying "mmm" when I am finished.

Another infringement on his privacy is his need to use a urinal at night. Waking from a sound sleep, which has been partially induced by medication, makes walking to the bathroom with unsteady legs a bit risky. His lack of awareness of just how one uses a urinal surprised me at first, but it shouldn't. This is Alzheimer's. My real problem is helping to support this big sleepy man and not let him fall, while he figures it all out. How would I ever get him up if he fell? We stay at the bedside. In case he falls, hopefully at least part of him would fall into bed! My very kind neighbor, George, says I may call him any time. So far I have not had to do that.

Dave has a new compulsion, that of changing his slacks and shirts. Several times a day he goes into his room and comes out a new man. Often he thinks we are going out, and he needs to look better. Sometimes he is too warm, or too cool, and selects something he thinks will be more comfortable, only to find, after a short time, that he has warmed up, or cooled off, and must go through the same routine again. At least it keeps him busy.

His latest habit is wearing his outdoor winter jacket instead of his sweaters, in the house. He does look a bit strange, sitting in his chair, reading or watching TV, up to his ears in that heavy jacket with its nice warm fleecy collar. When it is time to eat I have to cajole him into taking it off or it would forever be in the wash, the result of his becoming less adept at handling his food.

Losing touch with his beloved books is gradually taking place. I find him less and less often reading in his chair, and the books that once surrounded him are more and more left untouched on the shelves of his bookcase. He doesn't seem to notice that he is not reading, and I am glad for that, though I feel a sadness over one more plateau that has been reached. Along with the sadness is the need for me to fill that reading time with something else. The list of choices gets shorter.

One night at 8:40, Dave, out of complete boredom and disorientation, suggested that we go out for a ride and, "See what is going on." I suggested that he look out the window and see the darkness, that it was 8:40 in the evening and that it was doubtful that there would be anything going on that he would be able to see. He was completely mystified about its being evening. "If you say so," he said, but he continued to wait for the sun to appear. He wondered for some time about the strange sky and the lack of light. Finally he forgot about it and settled for a video, to my relief. That was the first time he had been totally disoriented as to night and day. Another plateau.

One night in February, with the family visiting us here in our own home, Dave got his jacket and suggested that it was time we went home. Another first, another plateau.

I reluctantly left him in April to go to Michigan for our grandson Mark's 30th birthday. Karen and Michelle shared his care. I did not tell him where I was going. For the first time in our lives I made up a story. I said I was going to see our friend, Nora. He accepted my statement without comment, thankfully. I felt enormously guilty, but it would have broken his heart to know I was going to see family without him. Trying to take him would have been out of the question, however.

He kept asking when I was coming home and was happy to go to the airport to meet me. But he didn't ask where I'd been or if I'd had a good time. He just said he was glad I was home. In a few minutes he had forgotten I had been away and was in his room all by himself, watching a video. I was glad. It canceled out my guilt feelings over having left him.

His care has become personal and complicated enough, however, that I have decided my trip days are over. I have made up my mind that we are looking down the long road ahead with no more interludes of R and R for me. They have been so valuable.

Added to that is the unsettling whisper of the thought that I am not sure how much longer I can handle things by myself. We have had three good months, but I realize that it is getting beyond my strength, and beyond the realm of safety for both of us. I know that, without a shadow of a doubt. His nights are becoming restless once again, and there is a feebleness that we have not coped with before which presents the constant possibility of his falling.

Are we again faced with looking for a nursing home? Where? How could I ever tell him? Could I manage those daily visits for however long it might be?

Those thoughts occupied much of my mind on into mid-April, especially at night as I readied him for bed: clean, medications given, eye drops in, pillow between his knees, bedding tucked around his thinning shoulders, windows open, light out, and my customary "Good night, Dear, see you in the morning."

Gwen Bibber Kimball

Chapter 30

OUR FINAL CHAPTER

Dear, dear Dave -

This is May, the year 2000. The rhodies and azaleas are turning our yard into a park again. You always loved this time of year. I think of you as I look out the window. I am writing our last chapter.

Since this intruder called Alzheimer's thrust itself into our lives I have wondered when, and under what circumstances I might find myself writing this, our last chapter. Always there has been the fervent hope and prayer that I would be here for you until you went Home. That would mean that I could be the one to care for you to the last, hopefully in your own home, and it would mean, also, that I would be the one writing this chapter.

God so planned it. How kind.

Although you did not regain your full strength after your bout with pneumonia you were able to return home. That was my joy. We had those three wonderful, quiet, gentle months together due to your medication changes. You lost your feistiness, and I tried hard to work around anything that could cause conflict. Our days were, for the most part, so very pleasant. We enjoyed a measure of compatibility I thought had been lost to us forever.

But you did lose ground slowly, so we made some necessary adjustments here at home to keep you safe. Your loss of your sense of balance worried us both, lest you fall and seriously injure yourself. I was especially concerned about the stairs leading to our lower level. Friends came and installed a dutch door at the head of the stairs. People of this generation seem not to know what a dutch door is, a half door with a finish rail on the top. Ours is done with a taff-rail. It is attractive, but even if it weren't, it was worth it. I never had to worry about that hallway again.

The second handrail on the stairs gave more security for you, plus an added assist for me. However, as you lost interest in your tools, screws, nuts, nails, etc., you went downstairs less and less.

Some rainy day I will start sorting all those things out and putting them back where they belong. Right now they are still where you left them on the work bench, along with other of your little projects you were no longer able to think through.

We took lots of rides those last months, didn't we? And I held your hand for many of those miles. It was the one way we had left to communicate. Your sentences were reduced to three words, maybe four -- not enough to express a complete thought, and when I could understand what you were trying to tell me, you had difficulty hearing and understanding the answer. We nearly always ended up in defeat. Hand-holding helped bridge that gap. Sometimes your hand would find my knee first, as if you were trying to keep in touch.

These are sensitive memories. I cry over them a bit -- not a lot because you are not a victim any longer.

And we had many cones of Mickey-D lo-fat ice cream, didn't we? You always forgot that they only had vanilla and you always wondered why in the world they didn't "get with it and start making chocolate."

I was thankful for all the videos the girls gave you for special occasions, especially those on World War II, and weather. You seldom seemed to tire of them, although occasionally you did lose interest after 10 minutes or so. Then I would wonder to myself, "What do we do now?"

Did you realize how helpless I felt when you would cry over your situation? I would hold you and try to stroke away your hopelessness. That seemed to be all I could do. I hope it helped.

The last few visits we made at Karen's house caused me some concern because of the need to step down into the parking area, from her front walk. You kept catching your heel on those two steps. I held your arm tightly and we did one step at a time. I was always glad when that was over. I knew I could not hold you if you fell, big fellow that you were. I could see us in a heap on the black top, looking old and pitiful, unable to help each other and calling out, "Help! We've fallen and we can't get up!"

Karen and I often played Rummikub and you would sit and watch longingly while we played. You wanted so much to be a part of it, but knew you could not remember how. I always had slight feelings of guilt at doing something without you.

During your last weekend it became apparent that you were having a reaction to your medication. You had become so rigid and your neck pained, and omitting the medication and trying Benadryl did not help. It only made things worse. You became very anxious and I didn't know what to do for you. I felt so helpless.

You were able to go to church on Easter Sunday. You looked absolutely impeccable in your gray slacks and blue blazer. Michelle took us to Karen's for our Easter dinner and we had some of your favorites: sweet potatoes, and ham with raisin sauce. But oh the trouble you had eating your dinner! For the first time it was a real disaster for you. The raisin sauce covered things for which it was never intended! I had to sort of fix you up a bit so you could continue. The next day your garments all went to Delken, the cleaner! Little did we realize that you would not wear them again.

Unknowingly we proceeded on to your last two nights at home. They were hard on you. You were increasingly uncomfortable and fast becoming helpless. You were unusually thirsty, and I knew each time I gave you water you would soon need to go to the bathroom. I also knew you couldn't get there, and you also might not be able to stand long enough to use the urinal, even if you could remember what it was for. How to manage? "Lord, please help," was my cry.

Those nights were hard on me, too. I was feeling tired, and so very old. I remember we cried together the first night and you said, "What can I do?" I pleaded stupidly, "Just please go to sleep. I am so tired, I just have to go to bed." You said you'd try, but in the midst of confusion and hurting, how does one just go to sleep? I guess I was too weary to be reasonable.

I know you forgave me for that. You did finally fall asleep about 2 AM only to wake at 4.

Before you went off to sleep I went to my room and literally fell to my knees and prayed, "Lord, you promised You would not give us more than we can handle; I'm 79. I can't handle this any longer and I need help." I did not realize at the moment that I was laying you, my priceless possession, upon the altar. I dried my tears before I went back into your room. I didn't want you to feel responsible for them.

The second of those two nights Karen came and stayed with us, but even the two of us couldn't handle your weight. We tried to help you to be comfortable, and then we napped when you napped, taking turns getting up for you. I think you knew you were in trouble because twice you asked, "Please pray for me." We held you as we prayed, and you said, "Amen" so fervently. You slept fitfully. Nursing Home again became an ominous threat.

The next morning Dr. Fiori said "hospital," for medication change and observation. I was so glad Karen and I were able to get you to the car for the ride there. You were still rigid but more comfortable, and of course I was vastly relieved that you were now to be in professional hands.

Our eleven-year-old-neighbor Byron was so helpful, reminding you of the steps and holding the car door for you. He carefully wrapped your blanket around your legs so you would be warm. You thanked him, and then told us you wanted him to come to know about God. We will do all we can about that.

After you got to the hospital they did an EKG and had you on the heart monitor for several hours. Do you remember that? Just routine, and all was well, they said.

New medications were prescribed. They took you to your room and I was aware of a sense of relief. I knew if your night was poor there would be adequate staff to care for you.

It was now evening. Michelle and Karen told you goodnight with a hug, and returned home to be ready for work the next day. As I left I kissed you and said, "Good night, Dear, I'll see you in the morning."

I slept. At 7:20 the next morning, April 27th, the phone woke me... dear Dr. Fiori. "I have bad news, Gwen. David had a massive coronary while waiting for his breakfast. His chin dropped onto his chest and he was gone."

My response, I think, was "Oh my goodness." I cannot possibly describe my jumbled emotions: grief, relief, joy, thanksgiving, shock, peace. Our battle with ugly Alzheimer's was over, sooner than either of us had expected. We will never know what we were spared. A gracious God, for reasons of His own, never took us there.

I called the girls. Michelle took me to the hospital where Dr. Fiori had waited. He went with us into your room, and then excused himself for our private time with you. You really weren't there. Only your poor thin, tired house was there. How obvious and comforting that was. We prayed and thanked God for the end of our struggle.

Dr. Fiori stayed while I signed papers, and then he walked with us to the door. A handshake could not express our appreciation and devotion to this uncommon doctor who had so endeared himself to us with his uncommon care. A heart-felt embrace seemed to be what I needed to give him, from both you and me. He received it graciously.

The family came, Midgie arriving that day all the way from Michigan. Grandson Michael and his wife Nadell came from New York. Grandson Mark, his wife Kristine, and great granddaughter Abi were in Europe and unable to be with us until later.

We made arrangements. People sent food, flowers and cards. Memorial gifts came for the new Executive Director's fund of Community Chaplain Service.

We had victorious visiting hours at the Funeral Home. You were in your gray suit with your 50th Anniversary tie and kerchief. You looked so scholarly, and so at peace. Many people came. One young man said he had never been to a Christian wake before and he had not expected to witness so much joy and peace.

We also had a Memorial Service at Mullein Hill Church. Pastor Ken led the service, Adele played. David Schaffer read II Cor. 5:1-8 from the Living Bible. We sang "Blessed Assurance'" in memory of your commitment to Jesus as a small boy, age 7, and in memory of Larry Wetzell, whose singing with us that morning so long ago gave you your vision for the Nursing Home one-on-one ministry. Your three daughters paid tribute, along with Walt Dryer and Glenn Havumaki. Roger and Mark sang, "There is a Saviour," and Mark sang, "People Need The Lord."

I paid tribute to you, my husband, with a mixture of pride, joy, sadness, and thanksgiving, you whose passing had left me with a huge vacancy, both at home and in my heart. Yet, I am quietly satisfied. God does hear His children when they cry for help, only He says, "I'll do it my way."

Pastor Ken spoke so lovingly of your person, your life, your service. He closed by singing, "Finally Home," followed by the congregation singing with him, "O That Will Be Glory

For Me." You would have loved it. It all spoke of the victory that is in Jesus.

Again, many people came -- but perhaps you know all about this. Were you privileged to see and hear all that I've told you? We can only speculate on that.

As I faced leaving you for the last time I knelt and laid my head on your shoulder. I said what I had said for many months of nights as I had tucked you into bed.

"Good night, Dear, I'll see you in the Morning."

EPILOGUE

Post-Alzheimer's Syndrome. Is there such a medical term? If not, there should be, at least for caregivers. I am not ready, nor am I able, to follow the suggestions of friends that I can now "get back to dwelling on days with happier memories." Strangely enough, some of my happiest memories reside right here in this time and place. I cannot leave them so quickly.

I feel I am confined to a time warp composed of Dave, Alzheimer's and me, plus all of the special people who shared our stormy experience. The many days, months, and years of Dave's illness, with their own vivid memories, seem to need time for scrutiny and reflection just now. It is too soon to let them fade. Their conclusion was too blessed and poignant, too timely and too compassionate, to close the book merely because the formalities of funeral and memorial service are over.

Those formalities indeed are over, but how does one go about putting aside the events, some pleasant, some difficult, without dwelling on the very positive messages they bear? I cried my tears and did my grieving over a long period of time. I no longer have great need of that, but I do need time to ponder.

I now realize I was literally driving myself at the end of Dave's life. I was doing what had to be done, in spite of the fact that I could no longer do it. Unreal paradox. One of the most comforting things I do these days is sit quietly and revel in gratitude that those days are past, those days of ever pressing on and on until Dave's light was out and his door was closed for the night. The relief is overwhelming. I was so sure that I could do it. Dr. Fiori was wise to ask that question even though my response was always in the affirmative. But I am left with the conclusion that feeling driven, as is the experience of Alzheimer's caregivers, masks good judgment. Caregivers, beware.

I wonder if that post-Alzheimer's syndrome to which I rather facetiously refer is a period of time necessary for a weaning process from the stark realities of those days and years. Those realities, and the realities of Dave's final days are realities I need to ponder for awhile; time to ponder Dave's ambush by this ugly illness, and his deliverance; time to allow the former memories to be healed by the latter. I need to remember our storm and let those memories abate as I focus on the Master of that storm -- He who heard me as I cried out to

Him by my bedside on that Monday night. As I ponder these events, I find I am slowly leaving my post-Alzheimer's syndrome time warp behind me.

As it fades I am experiencing an increased awareness of the reality of the One who is always waiting to be to us what He most desires to be, a personal God, a Father who sees us, knows us, and cares about our needs. Never before have I been so aware of the privilege of this relationship with the great God of the Universe. And wonder of wonders, He invites me to call Him Father, of all things!

This One, who programmed the creation of the incredible world we inhabit, also programmed the home-going of one of his children, my Dave, with such timeliness that it nearly took my breath away. In spite of the void it created, there isn't a detail I would change.

He who had lost nearly all his ability to care for himself, had lost recognition of nearly all of his family and friends, had lost awareness of his beloved books, had nearly lost sight of Heaven, had the personal attention of his Father who said, "Enough is enough, David. Come home now." I am still overwhelmed at God's immediate attentiveness to us. Dave is no longer a six foot 180 pound two-year-old.

This, then, is where my focus is for now, and I must express a final thank-you to Gloria Gaither for her reminder that we should build our altars in places where God has met us. My altar is by my bedside, the place where God met us on that Monday night. This is where I kneel in silence for now.

I don't know how long I will need to worship here, and remember, and heal. No matter. My heart and I are at one in this need to linger yet a while at this special place. Our Alzheimer's experience will take its rightful place in our history in good time, and then I shall recall our other days.

At the same time I must redefine who I am, all by myself. Having been part of a team for 58+ years leaves me needing to become acquainted with just me. After all, I was only 20, back there. Out of all those intervening years there must be clues left to indicate to me who I am and what I am about, for the remainder of my life.

But before those things clutter the scene I shall linger a little longer at that very special place where God met us.

****

Eight months have passed. It is now mid-December. It has taken that long for me to recover from Alzheimer's and get in touch with grief. I have just cried my first tears of quiet, comforting sweet sadness for the Dave who was, the Dave I once knew, the Dave who disappeared so mysteriously from before my very eyes.

I can now recall this one with whom I shared that whole-hearted love, whole-hearted energy, and whole-hearted purpose and I can cry in memory of that. The tears are brief and gentle, like a sudden shower on an otherwise sunny day, and when the shower passes it leaves no clouds. Only gratitude remains each time, gratitude that healing does take place in its time, and gratitude that Dave is safe Home.

Gwen Bibber Kimball is available for personal appearances and speaking engagements. To contact Gwen, write:

Gwen Bibber Kimball
C/O Advantage Books
PO Box 160847
Altamonte Springs, FL 32716

To order additional copies of this or other books
call our toll free ordering line: 1-888-383-3110

or

visit our online bookstore at:
www.advantagebookstore.com

Advantage
BOOKS

Longwood, Florida, USA

"we bring dreams to life"™
www.advbooks.com